The Complete Idiot's Reference Card

Calories Burned By Activity

The more you weigh, the more calories you burn performing any exercise because your extra weight forces you to work harder. The following chart shows how some popular sports and activities compare when it comes to burning up calories.

Activity	Calories Used Per Minute			
	120 lbs.	140 lbs.	160 lbs.	180 lbs.
Cycling (10 mph)	5.5	6.4	7.3	8.2
Dancing (aerobic)	7.4	8.6	9.8	11.1
Dancing (social)	2.9	3.3	3.7	4.2
Gardening	5.0	5.9	6.7	7.5
Hiking	4.5	5.2	6.0	6.7
Jogging	9.3	10.8	12.4	13.9
Running	11.4	13.2	15.1	17.0
Sitting quietly	1.2	1.3	1.5	1.7
Skating	5.9	6.9	7.9	8.8
Swimming, moderate	7.8	9.0	10.3	11.6
Tennis	6.0	6.9	7.9	8.9
Walking	6.5	7.6	8.7	9.7
Weight Training	6.6	7.6	8.7	9.8

Reprinted with permission from the American Council on Exercise (ACE) from ACE Fit Facts

Non-fattening Diversions

Here are some things you can do with yourself instead of eating. When you're tempted to eat out of boredom, loneliness, or frustration, go over the list and pick out an alternative activity.

- ➤ Have a manicure or pedicure
- ➤ Set up a fish tank
- ➤ Rent a movie
- ➤ Take a short train or bus ride
- ➤ Sign up for a class: yoga, low-fat cooking, art history
- ➤ Volunteer at a local hospital or community center
- ➤ Visit an art gallery
- ➤ Go for a make-up demonstration in a department store
- ➤ Read a new magazine
- ➤ Get a new hair style
- ➤ Browse in a bookstore or library
- ➤ Set up a budget
- ➤ Build a dollhouse or a doghouse
- ➤ Attend a museum lecture
- ➤ Get a massage
- ➤ Go to a park
- ➤ Buy a bouquet of fresh flowers
- ➤ Take a walk anywhere

Affirmations for Getting to a Healthy Weight

To use an affirmation, you simply have to read it and repeat it to yourself. Many people read affirmations early in the day and again at the end of the day. Some carry their favorite affirmations in their wallets as a reminder.

- ➤ I'm getting healthy
- ➤ My diet is becoming more balanced
- ➤ I can lose weight
- ➤ I'm reaching my goals
- ➤ I will be successful
- ➤ My life is changing for the better
- ➤ I can wait as long as it takes
- ➤ I enjoy exercising my body
- ➤ I can say no to destructive behavior
- ➤ I feel positive
- ➤ I'm getting there
- ➤ I'll get what I want
- ➤ I enjoy being healthier
- ➤ I'm proud of myself
- ➤ I'm in control of my health
- ➤ I have choices
- ➤ I can do it
- ➤ I'm excited about losing weight

alpha
books

What's in a Serving?

Bread, Cereal, Rice, and Pasta Group
One serving from this group provides about 80 calories.
- ➤ 1 slice of any type of bread
- ➤ ½ English muffin
- ➤ ½ small bagel
- ➤ ½ small (6-inch) pita bread
- ➤ ½ hamburger or frankfurter bun
- ➤ 1 small (6-inch) tortilla
- ➤ 1 small (2½ inch diam.) roll or biscuit
- ➤ 1 ounce of ready-to-eat cereal (This amount varies with the type of cereal, from ¼ cup Grape Nuts to about ¾ cup bran flakes to about 2½ cups puffed cereal.)
- ➤ ½ cup cooked cereal, rice, or pasta
- ➤ ½ cup corn, peas, potatoes, winter squash, legumes, or other starchy vegetable

Vegetable Group
One serving from this group provides about 25 calories.
- ➤ 1 cup of raw leafy green vegetables such as spinach, kale, romaine lettuce
- ➤ ½ cup of any other vegetables, cooked or chopped raw
- ➤ ¾ cup of vegetable juice
- ➤ Starchy vegetables such as corn, peas, potatoes, winter squash, and legumes are counted in the Bread Group

Fruit Group
One serving from this group provides about 60–80 calories.
- ➤ 1 medium apple, banana, orange, or other fruit
- ➤ 1 cup strawberries, blueberries, raspberries
- ➤ ½ grapefruit
- ➤ ½ mango
- ➤ ½ cup chopped, cooked, or canned fruit
- ➤ 7 dried apricot halves
- ➤ 10 cherries
- ➤ 10 grapes
- ➤ 3 prunes
- ➤ 2 Tbsp. raisins
- ➤ ¾ cup of fruit juice

Meat, Poultry, Fish, Dry Beans, Eggs, and Nuts
One serving from this group provides from about 150–250 calories. 2 tablespoons of peanut butter is equivalent to 1 ounce of meat and contributes 200 calories.
- ➤ 2 to 3 ounces of cooked lean meat, poultry, or fish
- ➤ 1 to 1½ cups cooked dry beans
- ➤ 1 to 1½ cups tofu
- ➤ 2 to 3 eggs

Milk, Yogurt, and Cheese Group
One serving from this group provides about 150–200 calories. Reduced-fat and skim milk dairy products may provide fewer calories.
- ➤ 1 cup milk or yogurt
- ➤ 1½ ounces of natural cheese such as cheddar, blue, brie, feta, gouda, mozzarella
- ➤ ½ cup ricotta cheese
- ➤ ⅓ cup grated Parmesan or Romano cheese
- ➤ 2 ounces process cheese (2 slices or "singles")

Fats
1 teaspoon of fat from butter, margarine, or vegetable oil provides about 35–40 calories and 4–5 grams of fat.

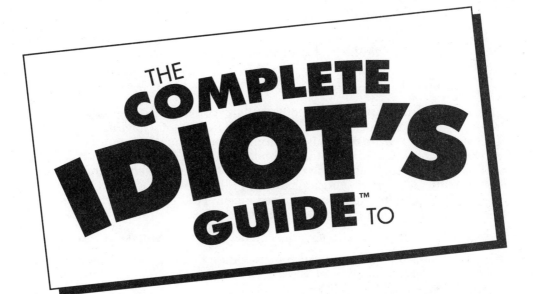

THE COMPLETE IDIOT'S GUIDE™ TO

Losing Weight

by Susan McQuillan, M.S., R.D.,
with Edward Saltzman, M.D.

alpha
books

A Division of Macmillan Reference USA
1633 Broadway, 8th Floor, New York NY 10019

This book is dedicated to my mother, Irene, who never told me I couldn't eat but always told me to hold in my stomach, to Margot, for helping me believe deep down, and to David, for daily reconstruction.

Macmillan Publishing books may be purchased for business or sales promotional use. For information please write: Special Markets Department, Macmillan Publishing USA, 1633 Broadway, New York, NY 10019.

International Standard Book Number: 0-02-862113-1
Library of Congress Catalog Card Number: 97-80967

99 98   8 7 6 5 4 3 2

Interpretation of the printing code: the rightmost number of the first series of numbers is the year of the book's printing; the rightmost number of the second series of numbers is the number of the book's printing. For example, a printing code of 98-1 shows that the first printing occurred in 1998.

Printed in the United States of America

Contents at a Glance

Part 1: The Truth About Weight Control   **1**

  1   Weight Loss: Fact and Fiction   3
      The truth about what it really means to be overweight.

  2   Why You're Weighty   13
      How you got to be a heavyweight, and why it's so hard to lose
      weight once you've put it on.

  3   The Cards You're Dealt   25
      How friends, family, and family history affect your weight.

  4   Heavy Thoughts   35
      Overcoming negative thinking and emotions that prevent you
      from having a healthier relationship with food.

Part 2: So Many Ways to Lose   **45**

  5   The Good, the Bad, and the Ugly   47
      Evaluating diet strategies, past and present.

  6   The Scoop on Group Weight-Loss Programs   59
      What programs are available for guidance and support, and
      how to know if a group is right for you.

  7   For Do-It-Yourselfers   67
      Setting yourself up to lose weight on your own.

Part 3: Small Steps You Can Take Right Now   **79**

  8   Kick-Start Your Personal Plan   81
      Starting off slow and setting weight goals.

  9   Dear Diary...   93
      Keeping a food and exercise diary and using it to change bad
      habits.

 10   Ready, Set, Go!   103
      Figuring out an acceptable calorie range for your weight goals,
      and developing simple menu plans.

Part 4: Nutrition 101   **115**

 11   You Are What You Eat   117
      Everything you need to know about calories, protein, and fat.

 12   Non-Caloric Nutrition   129
      Getting the vitamins, minerals, fiber, and other important
      substances you need from your food.

 13   Take a Look at Your Eating Habits   139
      Learning to use the food pyramid to keep your diet balanced.

 14   Guidelines for Healthy Living   159
      Putting the U.S. Dietary Guidelines into practice.

Part 5: Exercise 101   **171**

15 Why Exercise?   173
How exercise helps you lose weight, stay fit, and prevent disease.

16 Exercise Options   183
All the different ways there are to get some exercise, indoors and out.

17 Move It!   195
Balancing your exercise program with aerobic and weight-bearing activities.

Part 6: Mind Over Matter   **205**

18 Changing Your Ways   207
Learning how to make necessary changes in your attitude and your behavior so you can lose weight.

19 Handling Your Emotions   217
Working through issues of self-esteem, anger, confusion, and stress that can get in the way of a successful weight loss plan.

20 Thinking Fit   227
Listening to yourself, finding help and inspiration, and recognizing the power that your mind has over your body.

Part 7: Your Personal Plan for Losing Weight   **235**

21 Your Menu for Weight Loss   237
Choosing the eating plan that works best for you.

22 The Low-Fat Kitchen   249
Shopping and cooking your way to good health.

23 Let's Cook!   261
The ONLY low-fat recipes you need for basic, everyday cooking.

24 No Problem!   269
How to handle cravings, snack attacks, desserts, parties, and other temptations.

25 Keep Up the Good Work!   277
Maintaining your weight once you've lost it, and whipping everyone else into shape while you're at it.

Appendix A: Calorie and Fat Chart for Selected Foods   283
A chart of common foods with their calorie and fat gram counts.

Appendix B: Your Best Resources   291
Organizations, books, cookbooks, newsletters, and magazines that can help keep you motivated.

Index   297

Contents

Part 1: The Truth About Weight Control   **1**

1 Weight Loss: Fact and Fiction   **3**

The State of Overweight 4
How You Get Fat 7
Why Is It So Hard to Lose Weight? 7
Here's to Your Health! 9
Dieting Ups and Downs 10
Fat But Fit 11
Who Are the Losers? 12
The Least You Need to Know 12

2 Why You're Weighty   **13**

Are You Really Overweight? 14
    Measuring Up 16
    Apples and Pears 17
    When Overweight Is Okay 17
What's Your Story? 18
    Fat Cells Never Die 19
    Diets That Didn't Quite Cut It 20
Eating Too Much; Moving Too Little 20
Everyone's Different 21
Are You Getting in Your Own Way? 21
Undoing the Damage Done 22
    Look Behind You 23
    Now Look Ahead 23
The Least You Need to Know 23

3 The Cards You're Dealt   **25**

All in the Family 25
Fit Kids 27
What About Those Obesity Genes? 28
Brain Matters 29
Friends and Enemies 30
You CAN Lose Weight! 31
First Things First 33
The Least You Need to Know 33

4 Heavy Thoughts   **35**

Mind Power 36
   Mind Games 37
   Picture Perfect 38
No Guilt, No Blame 38
   Whose Guilt Is It, Anyway? 39
   Forgive and Forget 40
What Do You Expect? 40
Eating Disorders 41
   Anorexia Nervosa 42
   Bulimia 42
   Binge Eating Disorder 43
   The Medical Consequences of Disordered Eating 43
   Treating Eating Disorders 43
The Least You Need to Know 44

Part 2: So Many Ways to Lose   **45**

5 The Good, the Bad, and the Ugly   **47**

Dieting Through the Decades 48
Mixed Messages 50
   Low Fat's Where It's At, or Is It? 51
   Calories Come, Calories Go 51
   Protein's In, Protein's Out 52
   Up with Carbs, Down with Carbs 52
   Who's Telling the Truth? 53
Evaluating Diets and Weight-Loss Plans 54
Popping Pills 55
   Over-the-Counter Diet Pills 55
   Prescriptions for Weight Loss 56
Alternative Thinking 56
   What's Your Mantra? 56
   Fasting 56
The Least You Need to Know 57

6 The Scoop on Group Weight-Loss Programs   **59**

Commercial Weight-Loss Programs 60
   Weight Watchers 61
   Jenny Craig 62

Nutri-System 62
Diet Center 63
Repeat Performances 63
Life in the Fast Lane 63
Just for Support 65
Overeaters Anonymous 65
Take Off Pounds Sensibly (TOPS) 65
How to Evaluate a Group Program 66
The Least You Need to Know 66

7 For Do-It-Yourselfers   **67**

Are You Ready? 67
What's Your Motivation? 68
Ready or Not 68
Assess Yourself 71
Habits Are Habit Forming 72
How Did You Get Here? 72
What Are You Eating? 73
What's Your Plan? 75
You're Not Alone 76
Any Problems? 77
The Least You Need to Know 77

Part 3: Small Steps You Can Take Right Now   **79**

8 Kick-Start Your Personal Plan   **81**

Getting Off on the Right Foot 81
Check Your Attitude 82
Be Prepared 82
Time for a Change 82
What Are Your Goals? 84
Not Just a Number 85
What Can You Lose? 86
A Step at a Time 89
Let's Eat! 89
Move It! 90
Get Psyched! 90
The Least You Need to Know 91

9   Dear Diary...   **93**

What Exactly Is a Food Diary? 94
How to Keep a Food Diary 94
What Your Diary Tells You 98
Breaking Bad Eating Habits 99
The Least You Need to Know 101

10   Ready, Set, Go!   **103**

How Much Can You Eat? 104
   Calculating Calories 104
   More Than Calories 106
Simple Menus for Success 106
   Learn by Example 106
   Menu Sampler 107
Keeping the Record Straight 111
Your Incentive Plan 112
   Nonfattening Diversions 113
   A Job Well Done 114
The Least You Need to Know 114

Part 4:   Nutrition 101   **115**

11   You Are What You Eat   **117**

Understanding Your Metabolism 118
What Is a Calorie Anyway? 119
All About Carbohydrates 120
   It's So Simple! 120
   It Gets Complex 121
   Faking It 121
Protein Profile 122
   Where Protein Comes From 123
   Protein for Vegetarians 123
   How Much Protein Do You Really Need? 124
Demystifying Fat 125
   Good Fats, Bad Fats 126
   What's Your Limit? 126
   Getting Fat from Fat 127
   Fake Fats 127
The Least You Need to Know 128

12 Non-Caloric Nutrition   129

You Can't Go Wrong with Roughage 130
   Insoluble Fiber 130
   Soluble Fiber 130
   How Much Fiber Is Enough? 131
Drink Up! 132
   Other Watering Holes.. 132
   When More Is Better 133
Getting Your Vitamins and Minerals 133
   Vital Vitamins... 134
   Minerals Are a Must 135
   What About Supplements?.................................... 136
Phytochemicals in Your Food 137
The Least You Need to Know 138

13 Take a Look at Your Eating Habits   139

Exploring the Pyramid 140
How Much Is Enough? 141
   What's in a Serving? 142
   What Does a Serving Look Like? 143
   Picture This! 144
Balancing Your Meals 154
Putting the Pyramid into Practice 157
The Least You Need to Know 158

14 Guidelines for Healthy Living   159

Eat a Wide Variety of Foods 160
Finding Balance 162
Grains and Greens 163
   Getting Fresh 163
   Getting What You Can 164
Cut the Fat! 164
   Look Out for Saturated Fats 165
   What About Cholesterol? 165
Sweet Stuff 165
   Be a Sugar Sleuth 166
   A Rotten Sweet Tooth 166
Salt Solutions 166
Go Ahead, Have a Drink! 168
The Least You Need to Know 169

Part 5 Exercise 101 — 171

15 Why Exercise? — 173

The ABCs of Fitness 174
  Off to a Good Start 174
  Finding Motivation 176
  Weather Watch 176
Exercise in Good Health 177
  Exercise Styles 177
  Healthy Body, Healthy Mind 178
The Meaning of Lean 179
Your Workout Schedule 180
The Least You Need to Know 181

16 Exercise Options — 183

How to Join a Gym 183
  Step, Slide, Spin, or Sculpt 185
  Fitness Instructors 185
  Gym Etiquette 186
What a Sport! 186
  On the Green 187
  Tennis, Anyone? 187
  Take a Dive! 187
  In-line Skating 188
  Down the Slopes 188
  Off the Charts 189
Dance Your Way to Fitness 190
Exercising at Home 191
  Buying Equipment 192
  Exercise Video Picks 193
The Least You Need to Know 193

17 Move It! — 195

All About Aerobics 195
  Warming Up 196
  Your Training Heart Rate 196
  Cooling Down 197
Muscle Up! 197
  How Strong Are You? 198
Cross-Training 200

Walk This Way 201
    Your Walking Style 201
    Walking Off Calories 202
Keeping Track 202
The Least You Need to Know 204

Part 6: Mind Over Matter   205

18 Changing Your Ways   207

Promises, Promises 207
Are You Hungry? 208
    How's Your Appetite? 209
    Emotional Appetites 209
    Know When to Stop 212
Old Habits Die Hard 212
    Modified Behavior 212
    Table Manners 213
Check Your Attitude 214
    Change Your Food Attitude................................. 214
    Have Patience 215
The Least You Need to Know 215

19 Handling Your Emotions   217

Are You a Compulsive Overeater?.......................... 217
    Take This Test 218
    Dealing with Compulsive Overeating 218
Nobody's Perfect.. 219
Excuses, Excuses 220
    Putting It Off 220
    Pointing Your Finger 221
Self-Esteem 222
Lighten Up! 223
    Name Your Stressor 223
    Managing Stress 224
The Least You Need to Know 225

20 Thinking Fit   **227**

Who's Your Role Model? 227
No More Fear! 229
   Fear of Fat 229
   Fear of Success 229
   Fear of Failure 230
   What Are You Afraid Of? 230
Help Is Here 230
Practice, Practice, Practice 231
   Get Positive 231
   That's Affirmative! 232
   Affirmations for Getting to a Healthy Weight 233
   Words for Change 234
The Least You Need to Know 234

Part 7: Your Personal Plan for Losing Weight   **235**

21 Your Menu for Weight Loss   **237**

Pick a Plan 238
Straight Menu Plan 239
Pick a Meal 243
The Open Exchange Plan 245
   How It Works 246
   Take It with You 247
   Fair Exchanges 247
The Least You Need to Know 248

22 The Low-Fat Kitchen   **249**

Read All About It 250
   Just the Facts 250
   Label Lingo 252
The Healthy Supermarket 252
   Pick Your Produce 253
   Down Dairy Lane 253
   The Meat Market 253
   Birdland 254
   Today's Catch 254

From the Freezer Case 255
Cruisin' Down the Canned Food Aisle 255
Get Your Grain 256
Taking Stock 257
Fully Equipped 257
Magic in the Microwave 257
All Steamed Up 258
One Good Knife (or Two) 258
Just Basics 259
The Least You Need to Know 260

23 Let's Cook!   261

Soup's On! 262
Salad Fixin's 262
The Main Course 263
On the Side 265
Sweet Stuff 267
Good Substitutes 268
The Least You Need to Know 268

24 No Problem!   269

Cravings 270
Snack-Size Solutions 270
Solution #1 270
Solution #2 271
Solution #3 271
Solution #4 271
Sweet Surrender 271
Fruity Treats 272
Healthier Baking 272
Special Situations 273
Travel 273
Eating Out 274
Fast Food 274
Celebrate! 275
The Least You Need to Know 275

25 Keep Up the Good Work!   **277**

When You Reach a Plateau 277
    Stay Calm 278
    Plateau Busters 278
Weight Maintenance 279
    What You Know 279
    Stick to It 280
    More Change 280
    Go Back 280
    Move Forward 280
Pass It Down! 281
The Least You Need to Know 282

A Calorie and Fat Chart for Selected Foods   **283**

B Your Best Resources   **291**

Organizations to Contact for Information
  and Support 291
Internet Resources 293
Reading List 293
    Books 293
    Newsletters 294
    Magazines 295

Index   **297**

Foreword

When I graduated from college with a degree in nutrition, my first job was as a diet counselor in a health spa. It was very tough work, much more challenging than I had imagined. I'll never forget trying to help the overweight mom who had an addiction to peanut butter or the teenager who couldn't watch TV without eating something. I learned very quickly that it wasn't enough to simply give my clients a sensible meal plan and a list of nutritional dos and don'ts. To help them succeed, I had to make them analyze their eating behaviors, keep them motivated, urge them to exercise, and most of all, help each one to believe that they were in control of their bodies, their weight, and their health. Of course, nutrition lessons about calories, nutrients, and metabolism were vital, but they were only part of the winning formula necessary for achieving a healthy weight—and maintaining it. That realization, in essence, sums up the message and power of this book.

Susan McQuillan, herself a veteran diet counselor, knows that while losing weight is about changing your body, the effort to do it really requires changing your mind. First, with the knowledge of which foods make it easier to lose weight. And secondly, by consciously deciding to stop behaviors that put on weight and adopt actions that help you lose it. Ultimately, weight loss is all about decisions; between these covers you'll find all the information and inspiration you need to make the right ones.

What you won't find in this guide are any fad diets, gimmicks, special products, or starvation strategies designed to give instant results. While such get-thin-quick schemes may take off pounds initially, the weight loss is nearly always temporary because it's impossible to subsist happily on restrictive meals, powders and mixes, or a single food group. Dieters inevitably return to their old eating habits, and the lost pounds usually come right back. If you've been on and off the fad diet roller coaster you know how true this is. You probably also know that fad diets can make you feel physically sick, tired, and otherwise miserable. That's because many diets deprive your body of a myriad of nutrients it needs to work right and feel good. As much as being overweight is dangerous to your health, following a bad diet has its own risks.

Some say there are no simple answers to weight loss. I believe that there are—they're just not the same for everyone. What works for a friend may not work for you. Finding your own balance of good food, attitude, and exercise is the key to reaching your weight loss goals. This book is all you need to do it.

Elaine Khosrova
Food & Nutrition Editor
Healthy Living Magazine

A Note from Edward Saltzman

When I was first asked to work on this book, I immediately had two thoughts. The first thought was, "Why hasn't someone written this book already?" After all, this series addresses popular topics, and what could possibly be more popular than weight loss? In the U.S. about one in three people is overweight. And at any given time, millions of people are trying to shed extra pounds.

And then I had my second thought—this book hadn't been written yet because a straightforward, easy-to-follow, and scientifically accurate book about weight loss is a really tough thing to write. There's so much information out there about how to lose weight, and thousands of entrepreneurs will gladly sell you their secret diet, pill, or potion. It takes a knowledgeable, talented, and dedicated person to separate fact from fiction and what works from what doesn't. Lucky for us, Susan McQuillan is just that person. You'll find that Susan has written a sensible, enjoyable guide. Even more importantly, the information in this book is presented in a way that will truly help you incorporate state-of-the-art nutrition into your own lifestyle.

If controlling your weight was as easy as eating a miracle food or popping vitamins, don't you think we'd all be the weight we want? Controlling your weight is a complex process, and don't believe anyone who claims otherwise. But you can do it. Like other complex skills, such as driving a car, success can be achieved by mastering one small piece at a time. And when all those simple pieces add up, voilà, you're complex!

Living in this world full of food requires a plan, and a plan specifically designed for you by you is the one that is most likely to succeed. Who knows better how you live your life? So when you read this book, take small bites and give yourself some time to digest the information. And then spend some more time figuring out how the facts and tips apply specifically to you.

Finally, as time goes on, re-read parts or all of this book if you need to review principles or need some new ideas. Be flexible as your life changes. We're looking for a way to "do food" for the long haul, not just to drop a quick ten pounds now and regain it in a few months.

This guide provides all the essentials for weight loss and weight control. Use it in good health.

Edward Saltzman, MD

Introduction

If you feel the way I do about dieting—Enough already!—then this book is for you. Losing weight is complicated stuff, and a weight loss diet isn't a long-term solution for most people. That's because diets only work for a little while—just as long as you can stick to their strict and sometimes crazy rules! Once you break the rules, the weight comes back. If you've been on and off diets most of your life, you already know that.

But diet isn't a four-letter word. It doesn't just mean a way to lose weight. Diet also means how you eat. This book is about designing a healthy diet that's part of a healthy lifestyle that will get you to a healthy weight. If you sense that the key word here is *healthy*, you're right. Losing weight is all about making a commitment to your own good health. *The Complete Idiot's Guide to Losing Weight* will help you do just that.

In Part 1, "The Truth About Weight Control," you'll find out that even though thousands of low-fat and fat-free food products are selling out in supermarkets, and even though we're more knowledgeable than ever about the importance of exercise and good nutrition, as a nation we're fatter than ever. You'll learn why that's true and what you can do about your own personal state of overweight.

Part 2, "So Many Ways to Lose," describes the many different ways people have tried to lose weight over the past few decades. You'll learn what works and what doesn't, and what you can do to help make a group or individual weight loss plan work for you.

When you get to Part 3, it's time to stop reading and start developing your own plan for getting to a healthy weight. "Small Steps You Can Take Right Now" includes instructions on how to keep a food diary and how to use the information it gives you to explore your eating habits and personalize your weight loss plan.

Part 4 is a mini-course in good nutrition. You'll learn the ABCs of vitamins, minerals, carbohydrates, proteins, and fats in "Nutrition 101." You'll find out what a calorie really is and what it means to have a metabolism. And when you finish this section you'll know everything you need to know about eating a well-balanced diet.

Part 5, "Exercise 101," covers the basics of working out and points to exercise options you may not yet have explored. Want to go for a jog? If not, take a hike! Or maybe you like to swim. If not, how about a game of touch football? The list of activities you can use to help you get to a healthy weight goes on and on. Tango, anyone?

If your eating habits are tangled up with your emotions, Part 6, "Mind Over Matter," could be the most important section of this book for you. Part 6 will help you explore the thoughts and feelings you have about yourself that play a role in your relationship with food.

Last but certainly not least, "Your Personal Plan for Losing Weight" can be found in Part 7. Here, you'll pick an eating plan that works with your particular lifestyle. Part 7 contains a supermarket shopping guide, recipes, menus, and lots of tips for living a low-fat life...and still living a life!

How to Use This Book

Like any book, this one starts at the beginning and ends at the end. To get the most out of it, it's a good idea to read it in that order. But unlike a lot of books, you don't absolutely have to start at the very beginning. You can pick this book up and read any chapter you feel like reading. You can flip back and forth between chapters. This is a reading book and it's also a workbook. Write in it. Keep records in it. Make lots of copies of the blank worksheets and logs so you have a good supply on hand. Fill in the blanks and add your own thoughts.

Extras

You'll see at least one of these four boxes on almost every page throughout the book:

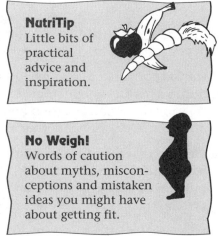

NutriTip
Little bits of practical advice and inspiration.

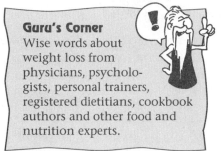

Guru's Corner
Wise words about weight loss from physicians, psychologists, personal trainers, registered dietitians, cookbook authors and other food and nutrition experts.

No Weigh!
Words of caution about myths, misconceptions and mistaken ideas you might have about getting fit.

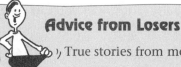

Advice from Losers
True stories from men and women who are winning the battle against fat.

Special Thanks

My personal thanks go to: Regina Ragone, who supplied resources, referrals, and special treats; Wendye Pardue, who (as always) supplied unfailing friendship and understanding; Joyce Rambo who lent an ear and an eye and kept me running; Larry Katzenstein and Julie Levine who kept those phone calls and e-mails coming; and Janine D'Amato who donated her Mondays and her many talents so this book could be finished on deadline.

My professional thanks to: Nancy Gagliardi for recommending me to write the book; Nancy Mikhail for hiring me and enthusiastically getting me off on the right foot; Lisa Bucki for superb editing and encouraging words; and Ed Saltzman, M.D., for giving it all the A-OK (and a few good laughs along the way).

Many people helped write this book, and I'm particularly indebted to every expert who contributed to the "Guru's Corner" boxes. I also wrote this book with the help of every successful "loser" who shared his or her weight loss story with me. A very, very special thanks to all of you.

Trademarks

All terms mentioned in this book that are known to be or are suspected of being trademarks or service marks have been appropriately capitalized. Alpha Books and Macmillan General Reference cannot attest to the accuracy of this information. Use of a term in this book should not be regarded as affecting the validity of any trademark or service mark. The following trademarks and service marks have been mentioned in this book:

ACE Fit Facts	Medifast	Ry-Krisp
Alcholics Anonymous	Metrical	Salatrim
Bran Flakes	Narcotics Anonymous	Saltine
Cheerios	NutraSweet	Shredded Wheat
Collage Video	Nutri-System	Slim-Fast
Diet Center	Olean	Sunette
Equal	Olestra	Sweet 'N Low
Farina	Optifast	Take Off Pounds Sensibly
Grape Nuts	Overeaters Anonymous	To Life!
Health Management Resources	Puffed Rice	Weight Watchers
Jenny Craig	Rails to Trails Conservancy	Wheaties
	Raisin Bran	Wheatna

Part 1
The Truth About Weight Control

Many people I talk to are confused about dieting and weight control. They want to know why it's so easy to gain weight and so hard to lose it. You're probably wondering the same thing, especially if you've been struggling to knock off more than a few pounds. This first part of the book is about the realities of gaining, losing, and maintaining weight.

These first few chapters discuss the "fat epidemic" that seems to have swept the country. You'll learn how you and a lot of other people got to your current state of overweight and what helps keep you that way. You'll learn the difference between "overweight" and "obese" and how to figure out which, if either of these, you really are. You may be disappointed to find out that there are no easy answers. But you'll be thrilled to know that there are solutions for every imaginable weight problem—including yours!

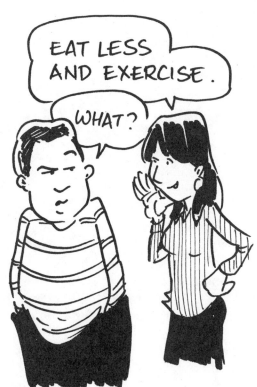

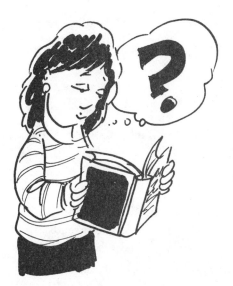

Chapter 1

Weight Loss: Fact and Fiction

In This Chapter

➤ What it means to be overweight

➤ Why losing weight is such a challenge

➤ How your weight affects your health

➤ Weight cycling: the ups and downs of gaining and losing weight

➤ Common traits of people who successfully lose weight

Are you feeling fatter than ever? Well, join the club! At last count, almost a third of all Americans ages 20 to 74 were overweight or obese. In real numbers, that means about 58 million people—32 million women and 26 million men—are carrying around a lot more fat than health experts recommend. Our kids are getting bigger, too. The numbers show that one out of every five adolescents is now overweight, and childhood chubbiness appears to be on the rise.

Health experts and other number-crunchers find these figures alarming because they're much higher than when we were last measured back in 1980. That was before we became a nation of fitness fanatics. After years of jogging, stepping, juicing, and eating low-fat foods, we're bigger than ever.

What's going on? Aren't we eating better food? Isn't everybody exercising? Obviously not. Whatever we're doing to battle the proverbial bulge isn't working for us; that's for sure. It seems we talk a lot more about eating well and exercising than we actually do.

Although it's true that diet and exercise play huge roles in weight control, there's more to this heavy epidemic than meets the eye. In this chapter, you'll learn what it means to be overweight, why it's important to aim for a healthy weight, and why it's sometimes so hard to lose weight.

The State of Overweight

Let's look at just what the experts mean when they say we're overweight or obese. These medical definitions are based on how far you are from "ideal" weights found on standard height/weight charts:

➤ **Overweight:** 10 to 20 percent higher than normal weight.

➤ **Obese:** 20 percent or more above normal weight with excess body fat. The official American Heart Association definition of obesity is "when body weight exceeds 'desirable' weight by 20 percent or more and when the excess weight is from fat."

➤ **Morbidly obese:** 50 to 100 percent above normal weight or more than 100 pounds over ideal weight or sufficiently overweight to have severe problems with health or normal functioning.

When you hear the word "obese," you probably think it means grossly overweight. There's no way it applies to you, right? Well, you could be wrong. Sure, you can be overweight without being obese but only if your extra weight comes from muscle, bone, or water. The truth is that most people who really need to lose weight are overweight *and* obese because they're carrying around a lot of extra fat. Most overweight people are also overfat.

Some doctors define obesity by percentage of body fat. Women with more than 33 percent body fat and men with more than 25 percent body fat are considered obese. There are several ways to figure out how much of your body is actually made of fat. You can jump into a pool designed for underwater weighing. This is probably the most accurate way to measure body fat, but very few places are equipped to do it. You can be hooked up to electrodes and have weak electric currents sent through your body. This method is easy for the tester but may be inaccurate in many circumstances. Not much point in that. You can be pinched with skinfold calipers—a method often used in gyms and diet centers—but don't believe the results unless you're being measured by a highly trained person using very good quality calipers. Because it's hard to get an accurate measure of body fat using any of these methods outside of a laboratory, they're best used as research tools.

Researchers use standards such as these to gather information and draw conclusions about the weight of the general population. That doesn't necessarily have anything to do with you. First of all, the concept of an "ideal" weight based simply on height is old-fashioned and doesn't really mean anything. Your age, your sex, your genes, and the state of your health all play a role in determining what your particular ideal weight can and should be. In fact, let's forget the word "ideal" altogether and substitute "realistic" or "healthy" when we talk about the weight you want to be.

There is a range of healthy weights for everyone, but your healthy weight isn't necessarily the same as anyone else's. (To see if you're in a healthy weight range, check out the weight chart in Chapter 2, "Why You're Weighty.") Your weight gain and weight loss patterns aren't the same as anyone else's, either. Just like your skin color and eye color, your basic body size and shape are predetermined by heredity. You can thank your great-great-grandmother for the size of your butt. Of course, you can probably thank the snack food and entertainment industries, too, because your basic body size and shape are altered by the types and amount of food you eat as well as how much time you spend doing nothing but watching TV! One thing's for sure: When it comes to healthy body weight, everyone's an individual.

No Weigh!
Don't think of your healthy weight as the lowest weight you've ever been or wanted to be, and don't compare yourself with other people. You have a healthy weight that's all your own, and it's determined by many things, including your individual body size and shape, how much fat you have, and which part of your body collects the most fat.

From time to time, government agencies collect information that gives us an idea of just how bad our state of overweight really is or how bad we think it is. The figures in Table 1.1 show the percentage of people surveyed in each state who said they are overweight.

Table 1.1 Percentage of People Who Claim to Be Overweight, by State

State	Men	Women
Alabama	26.2	22.9
Alaska	23.9	23.5
Arizona	21.0	19.5
Arkansas	31.8	28.6
California	24.8	24.3
Colorado	22.5	19.4
Connecticut	25.3	18.6
Delaware	28.1	25.2
District of Columbia	12.7	27.2
Florida	27.1	25.4
Georgia	23.6	24.6
Hawaii	22.4	18.0
Idaho	25.1	24.2
Illinois	25.5	25.7
Indiana	28.7	31.8
Iowa	31.7	24.7

continues

Table 1.1 Continued

State	Men	Women
Kansas	25.4	22.5
Kentucky	30.4	26.0
Louisiana	28.9	28.2
Maine	28.5	25.0
Maryland	25.1	24.7
Massachusetts	26.8	19.5
Michigan	29.6	27.9
Minnesota	29.0	25.2
Mississippi	30.3	32.9
Missouri	29.3	23.6
Montana	26.4	20.9
Nebraska	27.4	26.0
Nevada	25.5	21.1
New Hampshire	25.8	21.2
New Jersey	25.1	19.0
New Mexico	24.2	21.5
New York	28.5	22.6
North Carolina	28.4	25.3
North Dakota	30.5	24.0
Ohio	26.3	23.3
Oklahoma	25.7	28.2
Oregon	24.2	23.1
Pennsylvania	29.0	28.6
Rhode Island	25.4	21.5
South Carolina	29.3	27.1
South Dakota	29.6	26.3
Tennessee	27.1	27.5
Texas	28.9	23.5
Utah	24.4	20.6
Vermont	24.6	21.0
Virginia	29.2	22.0
Washington	27.5	24.6
West Virginia	31.2	31.1
Wisconsin	28.0	26.7

Source: Federal Centers for Disease Control and Prevention, Behavioral Risk Factor Surveillance System, 1993.

How You Get Fat

It's easy to get fat. Just eat an amount of food that contributes more calories than you're able to burn off as energy. If you've tried to lose weight before, however, you know it's not always as simple as balancing eating and exercise. Why? Because there are other reasons we get fat.

Fatness runs in some families. That could mean it's in your genes. But then how do you explain the fat family dog? It might not be genetic, but it could be environmental. That means you picked up your family's bad eating habits or sedentary behavior just by living with them. The type of food you eat, the times of day you eat, even how you eat—slowly, neatly, quickly, sloppily—are probably influenced, at least in part, by your parents, who picked up their habits from their parents, who picked them up from their parents, who...okay, you get the idea.

If you constantly ride an emotional roller coaster with cotton candy in your hand, you might have to get to the root of the problem before you can lose weight. How often do you eat when you're

➤ Bored?

➤ Lonely?

➤ Angry?

➤ Stressed?

➤ Rebelling?

➤ Sad?

➤ Anxious?

If you're usually pretty good about what and when you eat but still can't shake off the pounds, you might have to move more. Thanks to such modern conveniences as escalators and video players, we just don't move as much as we used to. We don't do as much physical work in our homes or at our jobs, and we certainly don't move much to keep ourselves entertained. As a result, we're not burning as many calories in our everyday lives as people did in the "old days."

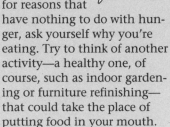

Guru's Corner

"I think one reason many Americans are overweight is because we eat so chaotically. We're skipping meals, bingeing, fasting, never feeling satisfied, and always looking for more food. As a nation, we need to rediscover normal eating and eating at regular times. We feel full when we eat a complete, balanced meal, but so many people aren't doing that anymore."

—Frances M. Berg, author of *Afraid to Eat: Children and Teens in Weight Crisis* and editor of the *Healthy Weight Journal*

NutriTip

Next time you find yourself chowing down for reasons that have nothing to do with hunger, ask yourself why you're eating. Try to think of another activity—a healthy one, of course, such as indoor gardening or furniture refinishing—that could take the place of putting food in your mouth.

Why Is It So Hard to Lose Weight?

Once you gain weight, it seems to stick like glue, doesn't it? That's because obesity is a chronic condition, just like diabetes or heart disease. It doesn't go away by itself, and it can't be treated quickly with a pill or a high-protein diet. There's no simple way to lose weight and keep it off.

Everyone's different. It's harder for some people to lose weight than for others. It's also unrealistic for some people to try to lose as much weight as others. No one really knows why some people gain weight more easily than other people and some lose weight more easily. You might have a family history of obesity, but if you're active and you make healthy food choices most of the time, you might never become dangerously overweight. On the other hand, if you have a family history of obesity and you don't exercise and eat right, you're more likely to get fat yourself.

Losing weight takes a lot of support from family, friends, and, sometimes, professionals. It's hard to go it alone. If your support system is weak, it's easy to give up and return to the old habits that keep you fat. Sometimes it's hard to ask for help, but surely there's never been a better time than now. If you don't have much of a built-in support system, the best thing to do is find a group that specializes in weight issues.

No Weigh!
Don't try to follow someone else's weight-loss plan if it isn't exactly right for you. You won't be able to stick to a diet that includes food you don't like, and there's no point in joining a gym if you can't find time to go on a regular basis. You have to figure out what works for you.

Sometimes we set our sights too high, and set ourselves up for frustration and disappointment. If you're very overweight, you might be better off aiming for "reasonable" weight loss at first, rather than making "healthy" weight your immediate goal. Take it slow. Even small amounts of weight loss can result in big improvements in your health. Losing just 10 percent of your body weight might be a reasonable goal for now. So if you weigh 170 pounds and your "healthy weight" is somewhere around 130, don't strive to lose 40 pounds at once. Aim to lose 10 percent, or 17 pounds. If, after some time, you've maintained that 17-pound loss, and remained at 153 pounds, you can try to lose another 15 pounds.

It's hard to lose weight, but everyone knows it's even harder to keep the weight off. Once we've gained extra weight, some strange force seems to bring us back to that state of overweight again and again, in spite of our best intentions. What's even more horrible is gaining back that lost weight—and then some! It happens all the time. This vicious cycle of losing, gaining, losing, and regaining is a direct result of dieting and just goes to show that most "diets" don't work.

If you want to lose a few pounds in a short period of time, just pick any low-calorie diet and stick with it as long as you can. You'll lose some weight. The problem is that it won't last. You'll get bored or you'll get hungry, and you'll go off the diet. When you start to eat normally again, the pounds come piling back on.

Diets are short-term solutions, and short-term solutions are temporary. The only smart way to lose weight and keep it off once and for all is to stick to one plan for a lifetime.

You have to develop your own personal plan and it has to be flexible, of course, and it has to make you happy. I can't tell you how many times I've signed up for tennis lessons because friends told me what a great workout I would get and how much fun I would have. The fact is, I hate tennis. I was always getting frustrated and dropping out of classes. What I do like is jogging and when I found a buddy to run with, I started going out three mornings a week. I actually look forward to it. The same goes for food. Some people like to cook from scratch. Others like to pull their dinner straight from the freezer case at the supermarket. It doesn't matter. The point is that you can't live by anybody else's plan, and you shouldn't even try. You need a plan that's all your own.

Here's to Your Health!

One of the best reasons for knocking off those extra pounds is that they could be hazardous to your health. Just being fat doesn't mean you'll come down with a killer disease, but obesity might contribute to the development of many chronic conditions. Here are examples:

➤ **High blood pressure (hypertension):** If you're obese, you have twice as much chance of getting high blood pressure as someone of normal weight. About 25 percent of all obese people have high blood pressure. If you have high blood pressure and can get to a healthier weight, you might be able to control your pressure without medication.

➤ **Diabetes (Non-insulin dependent diabetes mellitus (NIDDM) or adult-onset diabetes):** Almost 80 percent of people with NIDDM are obese. If you have NIDDM and you lose weight, you might be able to control your diabetes without medication. (Note: The other form of diabetes, known as juvenile-onset diabetes, is not related to weight.)

➤ **Heart disease:** Obesity increases the risk for conditions that lead to heart disease, such as high cholesterol, hypertension, and so on. Obesity might also contribute to heart disease independent of these other factors.

➤ **Cancer:** Obese men might have higher death rates from colon, rectum, and prostate cancers than non-obese men. Obese women might have higher death rates from gall bladder, liver, breast (postmenopausal), cervical, and ovarian cancers.

Almost everyone who is overweight or obese will gain some kind of health benefit from shedding at least some of their fat. This is especially true for people who have non-insulin dependent diabetes, a family history of diabetes, high blood pressure, or high cholesterol. At the very least, losing weight can help you feel better if you suffer from other conditions, too, such as gout, osteoarthritis, and certain types of sleeping and breathing disorders.

Advice from Losers

"My father and my brother both have diabetes, and so did my grandparents. But I still never thought it would happen to me. I used to drink at least three cans of cola every day and never even considered fruit for dessert unless it was strawberry shortcake. Giving up the sweet stuff has been one of the hardest parts, but I've discovered diet drinks and I work in a cookie or two every day. I've lost 30 pounds and my diabetes is now controlled by diet alone. I'm going to do everything I can to keep it that way."

—Cindy W.

If you have a medical condition, you should be under the care of a physician, and you should consult with your physician before you begin any weight-loss program. This is especially true of any weight-loss program that includes exercise.

Dieting Ups and Downs

Are you a cycler? If you have periods of weight loss followed by periods of weight gain throughout your entire life, you most certainly are. If you're a cycler, you probably go on a lot of diets. You lose weight while you're on the diet and then gain it back once you go off. Then you go on another diet, lose weight, and then gain it all back again. Up. Down. Up. Down. That's why it's called yo-yo dieting. At least one weight study suggested that people who go on fewer diets in their lives are better able to maintain their weight as they get older than those who yo-yo.

Some people say weight cycling is bad for your health and that it's better to stay at one higher weight your whole life than to suffer the ups and downs. The fact is that no one really knows if weight cycling is hazardous to your health. We do know a lot about the possible perils of carrying around extra pounds, so it makes sense to try to get to a healthy weight. Your goal is twofold: Stop yo-yoing and maintain as healthy a weight as possible by eating well and exercising as much as you can.

NutriTip
If you accept the healthy weight you can achieve by eating well and exercising regularly, you'll be able to break the destructive cycle of yo-yo dieting once and for all.

If you're overweight and frustrated by years of dieting failures, then your self-esteem has probably been down the tubes and back again. As you've lost and regained weight, chances are you've gathered a lot of emotional baggage along the way. If you've been trying to lose weight on your own and it hasn't worked, this might be the time to reach out to others who have struggled the same way you have or to seek individual counseling. You don't have to be alone with your weight issues. If you need help finding a group or an individual professional specializing in weight loss, start by calling one of the organizations listed in Appendix B, "Your Best Resources."

To stop weight cycling, you have to get off the dieting roller coaster right now. You have to lose weight and maintain your weight loss without going on any more diets. How do you do that? It's really quite easy. Instead of following every fad diet that comes along, you come up with that one-time, lifetime exercise and eating plan I mentioned earlier. And you stick to it. Along with that plan, it's just as important to form a solid support system. There are plenty of people out there, just like you, who want to help. All you have to do is ask!

Fat But Fit

If you're a control freak, you'll hate this: It's true that you can control the types of food you eat and the amount of exercise you do. But you might not have as much control as you want over how much you actually weigh. That number is often determined by factors other than how much you eat and work out. Your age, your individual metabolism, the number of fat cells you developed when you were young, and even your past dieting habits can all play a role in how much you weigh. You might be making every effort to weigh 110 pounds, but it's quite possible that nothing short of starvation will get you there or keep you there. Give it up! It's time you learned that you can't possibly control everything in your life and it's not very healthy to try.

Stop worrying about what the scale tells you or how your weight and body shape compare to someone else's. Think about it. Are you trying to do the impossible? Are you 5'2" and trying to look like someone who's 5'11"? Sorry. It won't happen. You're just not setting realistic goals for yourself. You can't stretch yourself to supermodel height, and you can't change your bone structure. You can't be reborn into a different family. When a friend of mine was feeling particularly short and dumpy once, a cute boyfriend said to her, "You look healthy and there's nothing sexier than that." It's true. The best thing you can do for yourself on a bad weight day is get off the scale, close the fashion magazine, stop daydreaming, and figure out how to get in your own best possible shape.

Fitness is the real issue here, not fatness. You might be bigger than you want to be, but if you're working out, chances are you're in fairly good shape and you might not have to lose as much weight as you think. Many overweight people have low cholesterol, low blood pressure, and other indicators of good health because they're fit. If you eat well and exercise regularly, your weight might not be a health issue at all.

Guru's Corner
"Diets make you think that if you just had more willpower, you'd be able to lose weight. If you stick to a restrictive diet for a few weeks, you lose weight and you think the diet 'works.' Then you start to feel uncontrollable cravings and you relapse. But that's because of the calorie restriction, not because you lost your willpower. It's not your fault."

—John P. Foreyt, Ph.D., professor of medicine and psychiatry and director of the Nutrition Research Clinic at Baylor College of Medicine, Houston, Texas

Who Are the Losers?

At least one out of every four of us is on a diet on any given day. In a never-ending attempt to get lean, we exercise, cut calories, pop pills, and even undergo surgery. In spite of our best efforts, there are more failures than there are success stories in weight-loss land. It's not the dieter who fails, however; it's the diet. People who lose weight and keep it off don't do it by following fad diets. They don't look for short-term solutions.

NutriTip
If you're an overeater, deal with your food habits first. If you're not active, more exercise might be a better first step. If you're an emotional eater, you might want to seek professional counseling as well. To lose weight and keep it off, you have to find the combination of strategies that works best for you, and stick with it.

Some people do lose weight successfully and they seem to have some traits in common. They follow rules, but mostly they invent these rules for themselves. They lose weight for their own reasons and not to please other people. Some successful losers join weight loss centers; some go it alone. Most important, they don't give up on themselves.

No matter what shape we're in while we're young, most of us start gaining some weight as we get older. In fact, the greatest gains often come in our 20s, 30s, and 40s. Our bodies change, we start burning calories less efficiently, and, very often, we're not as active. If that's happening to you, it might make more sense to switch your focus from weight loss to weight maintenance. In other words, don't try to lose enough weight to get back to where you were five or ten years ago. First things first! Just try to stay where you are for now. Use your best diet and exercise strategies to pull in the reins and stop yourself from gaining any more weight. Increasing your exercise is probably your best bet at this point because exercise helps boost your metabolism and build muscle, and that helps you burn more calories. The benefit will come as you start getting older but not fatter.

The Least You Need to Know

➤ One third of all American adults are overweight, but that means two thirds of us aren't!

➤ Dieting won't help you lose weight for good.

➤ To stop a life-long cycle of losing and regaining weight, you must stop going on diets.

➤ It's possible to be overweight and still be fit.

➤ To lose weight and keep it off, you have to make your own rules and then follow them.

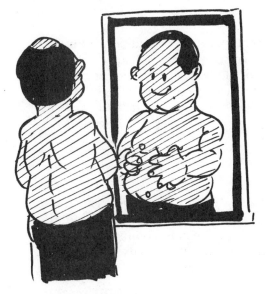

Chapter 2

Why You're Weighty

In This Chapter

➤ Formulas for figuring out just how overweight you are

➤ Examining your own weight history

➤ Why you can't compare yourself to anyone else

➤ What's stopping you from losing weight

➤ Learning from your past

I once read a survey that said 71 percent of American adults consider themselves overweight by at least one pound. One pound. I know a lot of people who would love to be overweight by only one pound. Wouldn't you?

As I read further, I learned that many of these "heavyweights" had no interest in dieting. Boy, was I relieved! A lot of them had already figured out that dieting to lose weight was a bad idea, and instead they were trying to adopt healthier eating and exercise habits. Way to go!

This chapter provides charts and formulas that will help you determine how far you are from your healthy weight. You'll learn some of the reasons why you might have gained weight and a few things you can do right now to start losing.

Are You Really Overweight?

When you're overweight, you can usually feel extra fat jiggling around on your body. Your waistbands are too tight, and there's a big bulge below them. When you're overweight, you don't feel comfortable with the amount of pounds you're carrying around. You can usually see extra weight, too. Look in the mirror. All the telltale signs of being overweight are usually right there staring back at you. Half of your total body fat is sandwiched between your muscles and your skin, and it's usually pretty obvious when there's too much of it.

The most accurate way to measure body fat is probably an autopsy, but it's hardly worth knowing at that point; is it?

NutriTip
The best weight charts give a range of healthy weights for different heights. That doesn't mean it's okay to gain up to the top of the range. The higher weights are for people with larger frames and more muscle weight. Typically, that means men and some very athletic women.

Check out all the ways you can measure yourself, and see just how overweight you really are while there's still time to do something about it. The most common measurements are the height and weight tables used by doctors, dietitians, and insurance companies.

The chart on the following page shows healthy weight ranges for both men and women. As you can see, there can be more than a 25-pound range for different people who are the same height. That's because two people who are the same height can have different amounts of muscle and bone. Men, for instance, often have more muscle and bone than women. If you have more muscle and bone than someone else your height and you weigh more than he or she does, then you're not necessarily overweight. The higher weight in each range probably applies to you. If your weight falls within the healthy weight range for your height and if you don't feel fat or unhealthy, you're probably not.

The higher you go above your healthy weight range, the more your extra pounds put you at risk for weight-related health problems such as diabetes and heart disease. A chart can only give you a clue about whether you're overweight. It can help you compare yourself to a "norm." But as they say, "What's normal?"

How fat you are depends on whose standards you're using to measure yourself. I hope that you're looking at healthy standards, not the ones defined by the fashion industry. Here's a quick formula that dietitians and other health professionals sometimes use to figure out weights for average men and women:

If you're a woman, start at a height of 5 feet and a weight of 100 pounds. Add 5 pounds for every inch of height over 5 feet. Then give yourself a range of plus or minus 10 percent of that total. Subtract 10 percent for a small frame or add 10 percent for a large frame. For instance, if you're 5'5" tall, a healthy weight is 125 pounds, plus or minus 12 pounds. Your range is about 112 to 137, depending on your bone structure and frame size.

ARE YOU OVERWEIGHT?

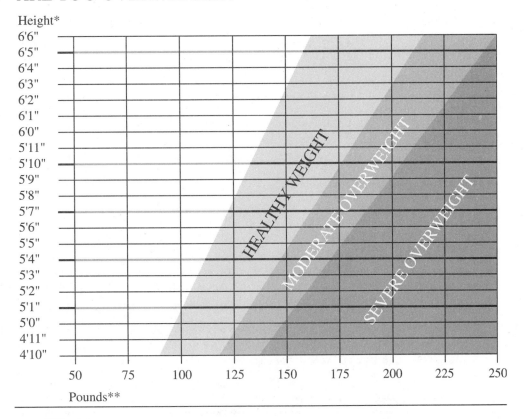

Height*

Pounds**

*Without shoes.
**Without clothes. The higher weights apply to people with more muscle and bone, such as many men.

Source: *Report of the Dietary Guidelines Advisory Committee on the Dietary Guidelines for Americans, 1995,* pages 23-24.

If you're a man, start at 5 feet and a weight of 106 pounds. Add 6 pounds for every inch over 5 feet.

There's nothing absolute about this formula, and it sometimes gives results that are slightly lower than the figures given in most height/weight tables. It doesn't give you a healthy weight range, just a single figure to work from.

NutriTip
No single chart, measurement, or formula can tell you everything you need to know about your weight or your health. If the results suggest that you're in a risky state of overweight, check with your doctor to see if you need to take steps to improve your health.

15

Measuring Up

Here's a more precise way to measure yourself. It's called body mass index (BMI), and it's a little more meaningful than a height/weight chart. You can refer to the BMI chart in Table 2.1 or use this formula to figure out your BMI more precisely:

$$\frac{704 \times \text{(your weight in pounds)}}{\text{(your height in inches)}}$$

For example, if you're 64" tall and weigh 145 pounds:

$$704 \times 145 = 102,080$$

$$\frac{102,080}{64} = 1,595$$

$$\frac{1,595}{64} = 24.9$$

If your weight is in a healthy range, your BMI will be between 19 and 25. A BMI between 27 and 30 is considered overweight. (A BMI of 26 is borderline. If your BMI is greater than 30, you are at risk of developing health problems associated with being overweight.)

To use the chart in Table 2.1, find the height closest to your own across the top and then move your finger down the column to the level of the weight closest to your own. The number where your height and weight meet is your BMI.

Table 2.1 Body Mass Index Chart

Weight (pounds)	4'10"	5'0"	5'2"	5'4"	5'6"	5'8"	5'10"	6'0"	6'2"	6'4"
120	25	24	22	21	19	18	17	16	15	15
125	26	24	23	22	20	19	18	17	16	15
130	27	25	24	22	21	20	19	18	17	16
135	28	26	25	23	22	21	19	18	17	16
140	29	27	26	24	23	21	20	19	18	17
145	30	28	27	25	23	22	21	20	19	18
150	31	29	28	26	24	23	22	20	19	18
155	32	30	28	27	25	24	22	21	20	19
160	34	31	29	28	26	24	23	22	21	20
165	35	32	30	28	27	25	24	22	21	20
170	36	33	31	29	28	26	24	23	22	21
175	37	34	32	30	28	27	25	24	23	21
180	38	35	33	31	29	27	26	24	23	22
185	39	36	34	32	30	28	27	25	24	23

Weight (pounds)	Height									
	4'10"	5'0"	5'2"	5'4"	5'6"	5'8"	5'10"	6'0"	6'2"	6'4"
190	40	37	35	33	31	29	27	26	24	23
195	41	38	36	34	32	30	28	27	25	24
200	42	39	37	34	32	30	29	27	26	24
205	43	40	38	35	33	31	29	28	26	25
210	44	41	39	36	34	32	30	29	27	26
215	45	42	39	37	35	33	31	29	28	26
220	46	43	40	38	36	34	32	30	28	27
225	47	44	41	39	36	34	32	31	29	27
230	48	45	42	40	37	35	33	31	30	28
235	49	46	43	40	38	36	34	32	30	29
240	50	47	44	41	39	37	35	33	31	29
245	51	48	45	42	40	37	35	33	32	30

Apples and Pears

When you look at yourself in the mirror, do you see an apple-shaped body or do you see a pear? If you have a pear-like shape because your body fat settles on your hips and thighs, you're in luck! People with pear-shaped bodies are at much lower risk of getting early heart disease, diabetes, high blood pressure, and certain types of cancer than people whose fat settles around their waist. If you can't quite tell which fruit you resemble, get your tape measure and use this method to figure out your waist-to-hip ratio:

1. While standing in a relaxed position, letting your gut hang out, measure your waist at its narrowest point. Write down that number.

2. Now measure your hips around the widest part of your butt. Write that number down, too.

3. Divide your waist measurement by your hip measurement. The result is your waist-to-hip ratio.

For a healthy weight, the ratio for most women should be less than 0.8, and for most men, less than 0.95. If your ratio is higher, you could be at an increased risk of developing weight-related health conditions. But there's hope! You can eat less and exercise to reduce your stomach fat and possibly reduce your health risks at the same time.

When Overweight Is Okay

If you suddenly wake up a pound or two overweight and you haven't been eating extra food, it's probably a temporary weight gain. Most likely, you'll lose it in the course of a week. You certainly have no reason to get excited or go on a diet. Everyone's weight fluctuates from time to time, even throughout the course of the day. It could be water retention, and it could be normal hormonal changes. If, over time, one or two pounds turns into four or five and starts leaning toward six, it's probably time to stop what you're doing and start paying attention.

You might be a few pounds overweight by the usual standards if your extra weight is muscle from working out. That type of overweight won't hurt your health. If you're overweight from excess fat, however, losing weight could be necessary for you to stay healthy. If you have high blood pressure, high blood sugar, or high cholesterol levels, losing weight might improve your condition. If you have a family history of heart disease or diabetes, you're more likely to develop these conditions if you're overweight.

NutriTip
Make good health rather than good looks your first motivation for losing weight. You'll have a better chance of maintaining a healthier weight throughout your life because you'll always be working toward a realistic goal.

Then there's the age-old question of what to do with the extra weight that creeps up on us as we get older. Although health experts say it's normal and okay to gain up to five or ten pounds as we get older, you might not like the direction your body's heading. My friend Linda says that when you get older, and especially after you have a baby, your butt and thighs are no longer separate body parts. She says they fuse to each other and become a single, mammoth unit. Getting them apart, she says, is almost impossible. She's exaggerating just a little bit, but I know what she means. It's a never-ending battle—even if you wage it at the gym—to try and stop those body parts from thickening and spreading.

It's crazy for most of us to think we should stay the same shape and size year after year. Still, many of us are fighting the good fight as long as we can. As we age, we lose lean muscle tissue. Exercise is the best way to hold on to some of that muscle and keep your body in its best possible shape. Besides looking good, muscle is the active tissue in your body where calories are burned. The more muscle you have, the more actively you burn calories. If you work your muscles enough with weight-bearing exercises, however, you might actually gain a little weight. That's okay because it will be muscle weight, not fat weight.

What's Your Story?

Were you a fat kid? Have you been fat your whole life or have you lost and gained weight over the years? Have you tried everything to lose weight, from crash diets to cabbage soup? A lot of theories out there discuss how your past diet and weight history affects your ability to lose weight right now.

For one thing, your eating and exercise habits are formed when you're young. Some of those habits change. (You used to hate vegetables and now you love them all, right?) The habits that have stuck with you so far are the ones you're not as likely to break as you get older. Those are usually the habits that get in the way when you want to lose weight.

Advice from Losers

"I've been overweight my whole life, ever since I was a baby. I've been at least a size 18 since high school. I never knew it, but we just ate too much food at home. I always had three pork chops or two hamburgers instead of just one and never thought twice about it. And I don't think there was ever an ounce of fiber on my plate! Now I have a skinny husband and he naturally has healthy eating habits that I've picked up, like drinking more water and eating more fruits and vegetables. I've lost 40 pounds and plan to lose a lot more. Still, when I go home to have dinner with my parents, I end up eating buckets of food. But now I plan it, and save my calories so if a day's worth come just from that one meal, I don't have to worry about it."

—Patty D.

If you're a fat baby, you won't necessarily turn into a fat adult. If you turn from a fat baby into a fat kid and then a fat teenager, there's more of a chance you will be a fat adult. Or you'll be a thin adult who has to constantly struggle to stay thin.

Fat Cells Never Die

You might be overweight because you have too many fat cells, or because the fat cells you have are size extra-large. Or you might have too many fat cells that are also too big. When a fat cell grows to about three times its normal size, it can divide and make new fat cells. How much fat a cell can handle before it divides varies from person to person. Scientists used to think we could only grow new fat cells during certain times of life, such as the first year and puberty. Now it seems we can grow them as adults, too. If you've gained a lot of weight as an adult, you may have added to your store of fat cells. That makes it harder to lose weight because once they've taken up residence in your body, fat cells don't go away. You can shrink the size of your fat cells but not the number.

If you suspect you have more than your fair share of fat cells, don't give up! I have to tell you the facts, even when they're a little depressing. It's my job. If you have too many fat cells, losing weight is more of an uphill battle for you than for someone with fewer cells.

Guru's Corner

"When it comes to weight loss, there's no such thing as equality of the sexes. Men are born with testosterone and the fat-burning machinery to lose weight quickly. Women are born with estrogen and the fat-storing machinery to gain weight quickly. Women's larger fat cells and pear-shaped bodies keep them fertile. When women go on a diet, their fat cells naturally fight back—and win!"

—Debra Waterhouse, M.P.H., R.D., author of *Outsmarting the Female Fat Cell* (Warner Books, 1993)

But it's not impossible for you to lose weight. You'll just have to work a little harder at it and be a little more patient. So what else is new?

Diets That Didn't Quite Cut It

Long before magazines and newspapers announced that diets don't work, many dietitians like me were trying to convince overweight people to stay away from fad diets. It's not easy. What can I say when my friend tells me that everyone she knows who follows a high-protein diet is losing weight and losing it quickly? Meanwhile, she's following my recommendation for a balanced diet and losing weight at what seems like a snail's pace. I reminded her that her diet was better both for her health and for long-term weight control. I also had to wait a while for the first high-protein drop-outs to report back and for the word to get around that it was no different from any other fad diet. One woman said to me, "It was a great diet while I followed it and I lost 40 pounds. But I just couldn't live without bread any longer." She went back to eating normally and regained the entire 40 pounds within 6 months.

No Weigh!
Beware of any diet that singles out a particular food or food group. You're not going to lose weight just by eating a grapefruit every day or by not eating pasta. You'll lose weight permanently on a balanced diet that provides just enough but not too many calories from all different kinds of foods.

Just about everyone who's ever been on a fad diet tells the same story. Meanwhile, it took my friend about two years to lose weight on her balanced diet plan, but two years later, she's still keeping it off, and she's happily eating whatever food she wants. There's more on that in later chapters, along with the details about different types of diets. For now, I just want to say that if you have a history of going on and off fad diets, stop now! They don't work. They're confusing to anyone who's trying to learn something about good health and nutrition. That's not what diets teach.

There are real biological reasons why severe diets don't work. When you go on an extremely low-calorie diet and cut back on the amount of food you normally eat, your body doesn't actually know you're on a diet. For all your body knows, it's being starved. It doesn't know when or from where its next meal is coming, so, being a smart body, it goes into "starvation mode." It slows down your metabolism, which slows down the rate at which you burn calories. Everyone's body has this natural survival tool. It's been handed down to us by cave men and women who used it to keep from starving to death when food was scarce.

Eating Too Much; Moving Too Little

There are all kinds of reasons why you're fat, and they go well beyond overeating. We've already discussed genes, fat cells, and rebound from fad diets. The bottom line to being overweight is that you're consuming more calories than you're working off. We can only spend so much time on theories and reasons. Eventually, we have to move on to solutions!

Everyone's Different

You might gain weight just looking at low-fat ice cream, while your best friend devours a double scoop every day without putting on an ounce. Sorry about that. Your metabolism is different from hers. Your attitude toward food and exercise is probably different, too. Your friend might also work her calories off in ways you never noticed. Maybe she takes the stairs when you take the elevator. Perhaps she walks when you drive. She might have more time to go to the gym.

Some people are naturally more active than others. In the normal course of a day, they move around more than other people and as a result burn more calories. I talk a lot and my head bobs around a lot, and I often joke that I burn extra calories just from moving my lips so much. It's actually true. Thanks to what's known as the "fidget factor," restless people can actually burn several hundred more calories than calmer types just from all the extra nodding and bouncing they do throughout the day.

No matter what your personality type, if you want to lose weight, you probably have to cut back on calories and move more. One way or another, a pound of weight always works out to 3,500 calories. To gain a pound, you must eat 3,500 calories more than usual. Likewise, to lose a pound, you have to eat 3,500 fewer calories than you have been. That means 500 fewer calories a day. You could also do enough extra exercise each day to burn off those 500 calories. Better yet, aim to cut out 250 calories and work off 250. It's easier that way.

> **No Weigh!**
> Don't be fooled into thinking it's somehow easier for others to lose weight and keep the weight off. Your friend might hate exercise as much as you do, but somehow she's learned to do things she doesn't like to do, and it's paying off for her. Life is tough. If you want to lose weight, don't let yourself off the hook too easily.

Are You Getting in Your Own Way?

It's easy to play games with yourself. The "if only" game is popular with a lot of people I know. "If only I had a lot of money, I could go to a spa to lose weight." "If only I could meet the love of my life, I would stop eating." "If only I had time to get to a gym...." Excuses, excuses! C'mon! Losing weight isn't about having enough money. It's about having the determination and motivation. People who go to the gym make the time, no matter what else is going on in their lives.

Another good one is the blame game. "I ate 45 cheese sticks because a customer called me stupid." "My brother said I was fat, so I ate a whole bag of cookies." "I overeat because my boss yells as me." Blaming is a way of giving up responsibility for yourself. It says that you don't have control over what happens to you. It says other people determine your fate and therefore your fatness. Blamers find it hard to admit that they're wrong about something or that anything that goes wrong is their fault. Sound familiar? Step aside! You're standing in your own way of losing weight and getting healthy.

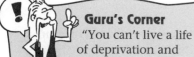

Guru's Corner
"You can't live a life of deprivation and denial, eating foods you don't like and avoiding foods you love. Don't overwhelm yourself with a lot of new diet rules. Eat what you like; just don't eat all of it! Commit to small changes at first so you don't get overwhelmed and give up."

—Ginger Patterson, Ph.D., R.D., Nutrition Director, The Wellness Center, Lee Memorial Health System, Fort Myers, Florida

Most of us could easily follow a few basic rules for eating well and losing weight if we would just take time to remember them. Some people don't eat often enough, so by the time they sit down, they're so hungry that they could eat a pound of elephant meat. Other people refuse to accept help, even when it's offered. If you answer "yes" to any of the following questions, it might be time to change a self-defeating habit:

➤ Do you look for quick fixes? All good things take time.

➤ Do you eat when you're not hungry? Think about why you're eating, and if you're not hungry, think about doing something else instead.

➤ Do you eat on the run? You don't have to sit down to three squares a day, but having some kind of schedule might help you improve your eating habits.

➤ Do you go more than five hours without eating? If you do, you're likely to overeat when you finally have a meal.

➤ Do you try to do it alone? People who enlist the support of their family and friends are more likely to be successful at losing weight.

➤ Do you give up just because you gave in? Everybody falls off the wagon once in a while and eats too much or indulges in high-fat foods when they're trying to lose weight. Forget about it. Just jump right back on the wagon. Don't look at every slip-up as a failure. You're a human and it's okay to act like one sometimes.

Undoing the Damage Done

It's never, ever too late to get fit. You're never too fat or too old to start eating better and exercising more. Only people with serious medical conditions have excuses, and even then, there's usually some solution.

If you've been on every diet in the book and still haven't lost weight, and especially if you've regained even more weight than you started with, you're probably very frustrated. I'm not surprised. For one thing, diets are exhausting. They take so much mental concentration and energy. When you're on a diet, your focus is on deprivation. All you can think about is food you can't have. Talk about negative energy! You become obsessed. It's no wonder you slide back to a state of overweight again and again. It's practically common sense to respond to food deprivation by overeating.

Look Behind You

Think about the diets you've experienced. Figure out what was wrong with each and don't make any plans to repeat it. For instance, maybe you were on a diet that limited you to 1,200 calories a day, and you couldn't stick to it because you were too hungry. You shouldn't try to routinely go that low in calories again. Maybe the diet was so high in fiber it caused excess gas, and you were in so much pain you had to stop immediately. You probably won't even be tempted to do that again! Next, figure out what you liked about certain diets and what you felt comfortable with. Perhaps you lost weight with a reasonable calorie restriction but didn't like the food you were told to eat. That tells you something. You can probably live comfortably on fewer calories than you're now eating, but they have to come from foods you enjoy. That shouldn't be a problem. As a matter a fact, that's what this book is all about.

> **NutriTip**
> Keep your food life interesting by experimenting with new foods. Try an exotic fruit you've never tasted before. Order something totally different on the menu when you go out to eat. Take a cooking class and learn new ways to prepare food. Look for low-fat cooking classes so you can learn how to prepare healthier foods.

Now Look Ahead

Along the way in life, we pick up lots of habits, good and bad. This is as good a time as any to start paying more attention to your eating habits. You know what you have to do. Ditch the late-night snacks. Find something to do besides eat when you're bored or upset. At the same time, keep eating some of those lower-fat foods. Keep experimenting with new foods. Your goal for now is to feel good and not guilty or mad about what you eat.

I always tell people who want to lose weight to throw themselves into the subject completely. I don't mean get obsessive. I mean use your spare time to learn all you can about nutrition and exercise. Read books and magazines, watch videos and television shows, and if you have access to the World Wide Web, search for motivation. Be discriminating about where you find your information. Be sure that it comes from a registered dietitian, a state licensed or certified nutritionist, a government source, a medical doctor, an exercise physiologist, or a certified trainer. For some reliable references in all areas of weight loss, check Appendix B, "Your Best Resources," at the back of this book.

The Least You Need to Know

➤ Your goal is not to be like someone else but to reach your own personal healthy weight.

➤ No matter how many times you've tried before, you can lose weight now.

➤ To lose weight, you have to burn more calories than you consume.

➤ Learning about good food and good nutrition can help you lose weight and keep it off.

➤ Some people lose weight faster and easier than others, but there's a weight-control solution for everyone.

23

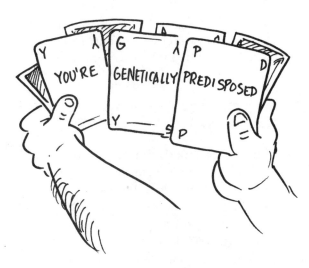

Chapter 3

The Cards You're Dealt

> ## In This Chapter
>
> ➤ What to do when everyone in your family is overweight
>
> ➤ Fat genes and mutant mice
>
> ➤ How your brain affects the way you eat
>
> ➤ Handling people who aren't as supportive as they could be
>
> ➤ Steps you can take to start losing weight

My mother recently said to me, "Well, if it makes you feel any better, I've always had big thighs, too." I can't say I felt better, especially because I hadn't even mentioned my thighs, but suddenly something became very clear. Money isn't the only thing we stand to inherit from our parents.

The good news is that you don't inherit fatness. You only inherit a tendency to become fat. That's good news because it's a lot easier to do something about a tendency. In this chapter, you'll learn how your family history affects your weight and how family members and friends can affect your weight-loss success. This chapter also suggests small steps you can take right now to prepare for a fit future.

All in the Family

Maybe you eat too much. Maybe you don't exercise enough. But you also may have inherited your weight problem from one or both of your parents. Does fat run in your family? If so, you have a much better chance of being fat yourself than someone with lean relatives. The real question—is fat in your genes or in your environment? Did you inherit a genetic tendency to get fat or just some bad eating habits? Likely as not, you got a little bit of both.

Advice from Losers

"No one in my family is thin. We're Italian, and food is a really big deal at our house. Of course, my mom's a great cook, and there were always huge piles of food on the table. When I wanted to lose weight for my friend's wedding, I started looking at low-fat cookbooks and recipes, including a lot of pasta recipes. I said to my mother, 'I bet we could all lose weight if you cooked this way.' She started cooking lower-fat foods and everyone lost weight—my father, my mother, and me! I lost 15 pounds over the summer. After that, I wasn't losing any more, so I decided to start exercising to lose 10 more pounds. It worked! I'm still pretty much eating and exercising the same way, and I've kept those 25 pounds off for 2 years."

—Joann F.

You don't have to fulfill your fat destiny. Coming from a fat family makes it harder to lose weight, but it's not impossible. If you live with your family and you want to start eating better, enlist their help and support. Figure out exactly what you want your parents or other family members to do. Do you want your mother to cook differently? Would it help if your sister stopped leaving potato chips on the kitchen counter? Think about the different ways your family unknowingly sabotages your attempts at better eating. Maybe all you have to do is ask. But no blaming! Your weight issues are your own. You just want to explain your goals to your family and ask for their support. Tell them specifically what they can do to help. Maybe they'll want to jump on the bandwagon, but they might not. All you can do is make suggestions.

Here are a just few ways families can cooperate to break old habits and introduce new ones together:

➤ Shop together. If everyone goes to the supermarket, everyone has a chance to pick out their favorite healthy foods and to remind each other not to buy junk food! (Check out Chapter 22, "The Low-Fat Kitchen," for more tips and information on shopping for healthy foods.)

➤ Cook together. Share what you know about low-fat cooking with the rest of the family.

➤ Serve food in reasonably sized portions on individual plates, rather than "family style," where serving bowls are passed and everyone helps themselves.

➤ In place of the after-dinner mint, take an after-dinner walk. That's right. The whole family. Together. Take the dog.

➤ Encourage family activities that get everyone moving. Set up a volleyball net, get everyone on a bicycle, plan a hiking vacation this year, or just throw a ball around in the backyard.

Fit Kids

When you were a kid, how often did you hear, "Clean your plate or no dessert!" How about, "Children in China are starving!" (as if eating your spinach would help them). Parents will say anything to get their kids to eat healthy foods. Sometimes these commands and insinuations also teach us to eat too much food and set a negative tone for how we view different types of food. Anything we're forced to do, such as eat spinach, becomes more and more unappealing, whereas something we're not allowed to do, such as eat dessert first, becomes more and more attractive.

If you're a parent, you might wonder whether to ever give in to your child's demands for junk food. Some parents forbid sweet and fatty foods, but others look the other way when their kid eats candy. If fatness runs in the family, you won't be helping your child's chances of staying lean by indulging his every doughnut dream. You also don't want to increase his desire for junk food by absolutely forbidding it. The best thing you can do is take a firm middle ground. Plan your child's snacks to include favorite treats. The key word here is plan. Teach your child that snacking is okay when it's under control by having a routine such as cookies and milk after school. Give your kids choices that include healthy foods, and let them choose the snacks they most enjoy. At the same time you're saying yes to healthy, planned snacking, it's okay to say no to continuous snacking in front of the TV at night or to random grabbings on the way out of the house.

Parents who use food as a reward or as a Band-Aid for hurt feelings send the wrong message to their children. The message says you can use food to fix what's wrong with your life. Wrong! If you eat when you have emotional problems, you probably got that message early. Now you connect food with love, so whenever you feel sad or lonely or hurt, it only makes sense that you turn to food for comfort. (For more information about emotional eating and what you can do about it, check out Part 6, "Mind Over Matter.")

NutriTip
Everyone in the family who's over two years old will benefit from a healthy and low-fat diet and a group activity plan. Kids and teens will pick up important habits they might follow their whole lives. Adults will stay in better shape and lower their risk of getting weight-related diseases.

No Weigh!
Don't give your kids large portions of food. Instead, offer them small amounts of different types of food, and let them ask for second helpings of their favorites. That way you'll teach your kids acceptable portion sizes—not to accept huge helpings of food as normal.

What About Those Obesity Genes?

In 1994, the news spread far and wide that obesity researchers had discovered a gene that, when damaged, causes mice to get fat. They named it the OB gene, short for obese gene. The OB gene is found in fat cells. Its job is to make a hormone-like protein called leptin that sends a signal to the brain that lets the mouse know when its fat cells are full so it will stop eating. Got that? Okay. Obese mice have defective OB genes that forget to make leptin or produce too little of it, so the signal to stop eating doesn't get sent. Oops! Twenty-five pounds of cheese later…you've got one fat mouse.

You are not a rodent, but scientists knew they could use the mouse gene to locate a similar gene in humans. And they did that. Then they tested mice to see what would happen if they were given leptin supplements. The mice ate less and lost weight. Leptin also increased their metabolic rates. Of course, the scientists were very excited and hoped to find the same results when leptin was given to humans. It soon became obvious, however, that obesity in humans is more complicated than in mice. For one thing, it involves more than a single gene.

NutriTip
Having trouble getting into your genes? Here's all you need to know: Genes consist of DNA (deoxyribonucleic acid). DNA contains instructions for your body to make different kinds of proteins. These proteins determine the color of your eyes, the shade of your skin, the basic shape of your body, and other individual traits.

Right on the heels of the OB gene came the discovery of another mouse gene. This one, called the "fat" gene, or CPE, controls the way fat is metabolized, rather than controlling appetite as the OB gene does. The thinking here is that dysfunctional "fat" genes interfere with fat metabolism because they interfere with insulin production. (Insulin plays an important role in helping your body use fat.)

Moving right along, we have the discovery of UCP2, a gene that activates a protein that "steals" energy from cells. The cells have to burn extra calories to make up for the energy they've lost. This brought speculation that maybe people are fat because their UCP2 is defective and they don't burn calories as well as someone whose UCP2 is in tip-top shape. Stay tuned….

Genetic discoveries are probably more exciting to the pharmaceutical industry than to anyone else. Eventually, scientists hope to develop new weight loss drugs that work by fixing all these damaged genes or compensating for what's missing so we can all lose weight. Other drugs will make the UCP2 gene work harder so your body will burn off more calories. Tests will be developed to predict genetic tendencies toward obesity while we're still young. Imagine the possibilities. Drug companies already have! One company paid about $20 million for a patent license on OB gene and leptin research. You can be sure that new medical treatments are coming down the pipeline, but it will be some time before we really know how to patch our genes. Scientists are still figuring out what genes mean, and then it will take time for appropriate drugs to be developed and even more time to test them for side effects.

Brain Matters

Did you know that your brain and body are in cahoots when it comes to what and how you eat? One is constantly signaling the other to communicate information about how hungry or full you are, how much food you're eating, and whether you want a salty snack or a sweet. Different foods, in turn, cause new and different signals to be sent back and forth between your brain and your body.

Your brain is your body's food control center. Hunger and fullness are registered here, appetite is controlled, and metabolism is guided by billions of brain cells known as neurons. Neurons communicate with each other by sending messages about your moods, emotions, and feelings, as well as physical hunger. Chemicals called neurotransmitters carry these messages from one brain cell to another and throughout the body.

Have you ever noticed that certain foods seem to throw you into different kinds of moods? Some researchers say that what you eat affects the balance of some of the neurotransmitters, such as serotonin and dopamine, that play a role in mood and appetite control. In turn, the balance of these neurotransmitters can affect the way you feel.

It happens the other way around, too. Certain moods might affect the type of food you choose to eat. Like many people, my friend Regina craves starchy carbohydrates when she feels anxious. She can't seem to get enough crackers and bread. When she eats these carbohydrates, she says she actually feels calmer.

Other chemicals in your brain and throughout your body influence when you eat, the type of foods you eat, how much you eat, and whether you're even hungry. Somehow they're always tied in to mood. You may have heard about endorphins, chemicals naturally produced by your body to help you cope with stress and pain. They make you feel better. Chocolate, ice cream, and other sweet and creamy foods seem to trigger the release of endorphins, and that's why some people think of these foods as "mood elevators." In turn, endorphins are thought to trigger cravings for these very same foods. That's one reason why it might not be such a good idea for some people to use these foods as mood soothers.

Skipping meals and overeating are habits that send your brain chemicals and body hormones into a tailspin and can ultimately cause you to binge. Add that to your list of reasons for eating regular, balanced meals as a means to weight control.

Guru's Corner

"Levels of the brain chemical serotonin, which regulates your moods and carbohydrate cravings, drop in some people during the winter months. If you suffer from mild depression, increased food cravings, and weight gain during the winter, you may crave lots of sweets and starches. These foods raise serotonin levels, improve mood, produce a calming effect, and curb the cravings."

—Elizabeth Somer, M.A., R.D., author of *Food and Mood: The Complete Guide to Eating Well and Feeling Your Best* (Henry Holt and Company, 1995)

Friends and Enemies

Losing weight takes a lot of determination, and a lot of support. When you look for that support, where do you turn? To your mate, your parents, your closest friends? They're the ones who can help you, but just remember one thing: They love you the way you are. They love you overweight.

No Weigh!
Don't let other people's personal issues get in the way of your losing weight. If your doctor says you need to lose weight, then you need to lose weight. Some of your friends and relatives might resist your weight loss just because it's a change, and some people have a hard time accepting any type of change.

Yes, it's completely up to you to lose your extra weight. The truth is, we all need help. We need people to pay attention to what we're doing, and we need a pat on the back when we do it well. If you're trying to lose weight, you're trying to be self-supportive instead of self-destructive. You want the people around you to help you make the necessary changes in your life.

If losing weight means you have to stop going to Sunday supper at your parent's house for a while or not eat as much of your mother's cooking as you used to, family members might take it personally and feel hurt. If losing weight means you'll be more attractive to other men or women, your mate might not be as supportive as you'd hoped. If losing weight means you'll soon be looking better than your best friend, expect some resistance from her. Everyone's used to you the way you are. Don't be surprised if they want you to stay that way. People might tell you that you look great and that you don't need to lose weight. They might have their own reasons for wanting you to stay the way you are, or they just might not be taking you seriously. Maybe they're afraid that they'll hurt your feelings if they agree with you.

Sometimes the people you most need support from will let you down. It happens. When it does, you have to be strong enough to rise above everyone else's issues. Most likely, they don't even know they're hurting your chances at success. You might have to be the one to point it out to them. They, in turn, might feel hurt. If you can muster up the incredible amount of courage it takes to lose weight, you can muster up the courage to stand up to anyone who tries to stop you. This will be a true test. If you want to lose weight, you might have to be a little selfish. That's selfish in a most positive sense of the word because it could save your life.

Remember, part of your goal is to stop worrying about what others think. You want to stop pleasing everyone but yourself. You're trying to take control of something in your life, and that means asserting yourself right now, no matter what anyone else says. It doesn't mean you have to stop caring about those you love. It just means you're starting to care about yourself now, too.

Learn how to say "No, thank you," and "No, thanks, Mom; I don't want any more mashed potatoes," even though you know she'll take it personally. "No, dear, I'd rather eat at home tonight," even though your mate is dying to go out. "No, thanks," even though your hostess will be insulted. If you can, practice what you're going to say before the situation even arises. Be firm and don't let anyone argue with you. You'll hear, "Oh, just this once" or "How long are you going to be on this diet?" Try to have your answers ready and don't give in!

You won't always have to say no to everything and maybe it will help to explain that. Help your friends and family understand that right now you're trying to break bad old habits. It's going to take a lot of work and a lot of positive reinforcement. Explain that you're not trying to be antisocial or impolite. Let the people you care about know that this isn't just another diet, but that you're trying to make big changes in the way you eat and live so that you never have to think about dieting again. Tell them what you need them to do and say. They might not know how to be supportive and you'll have to teach them as you go along. When you get the attention and support you need, remember to say "Thank you."

Guru's Corner

"You don't have to isolate yourself from social activities, but you have to stand firm. If you're going to dinner at your mother-in-law's, call her ahead of time and explain that you're watching what you eat. If you're invited to have seconds, simply smile and pass. This is your call; you don't have to give excuses to yourself or anyone else."

—Marjorie Jones-Laird, Ph.D., Psychotherapist, Ontario, California

You CAN Lose Weight!

I get into the deeper roots of overeating in the next chapter. For now, you know there are many reasons why you're a heavyweight besides overeating and underexercising. You might have inherited fat genes from your family. They might have had a bad influence on your eating habits when you were young. What can you do with this information? First of all, you can release yourself from some of the responsibility you take for your weight. You can stop blaming yourself, but you can't turn that blame and responsibility over to someone else. No one else can lose weight for you. Instead, use what you know about your family's role to put your weight problem in perspective. Armed with all this knowledge, you can start getting serious about losing weight once and for all.

Advice from Losers

"I gained about 30 pounds when I quit smoking and didn't have a clue what to do about it. One day I was watching my brother eat, and it reminded me of a *National Geographic* special about a hyena feasting at a zebra kill. It was quick and it was messy. When I realized my eating habits weren't much different, I consciously slowed down and started paying more attention to everything I was putting in my mouth. I started to enjoy my food more, and I discovered that the slower I ate, the less I ate. That's probably why I was able to lose the weight in less than a year's time. I still eat slowly and carefully, and I think that's one of the reasons, along with exercise, that I've been able to keep the weight off for more than ten years."

—Jeff K.

No matter what else is going on in your life right now, take a little time to start laying the groundwork for a healthier future. Look over this list. Pick something that's easy for you to do right now or at least think about right now:

➤ Start setting short-term goals. Instead of worrying about where you want your weight to be in four months, decide where you can reasonably expect it to be in, say, four weeks. A good short-term goal is to lose three to five pounds in four weeks. Be specific, but give yourself a little leeway.

➤ Set even shorter-term goals. Shorter-term goals help you reach your short-term goals. You've heard the expression, "a day at a time." This is what it means. Every day you have a goal just for that day. If you know you're going to the gym, today's goal could be to stay on the treadmill five minutes longer. You don't have to commit to that extra five minutes tomorrow. It's just your goal for today. Tomorrow you might decide to sit down and have bran flakes and banana slices for breakfast instead of your usual Pop Tart in the car.

➤ Think about what you want. To reach your goals, you have to be clear and honest with yourself about what you're willing to do to get there. Are you ready to lose weight? Are you willing to make the changes necessary for you to lose weight? Do you want to count calories and fat grams at every meal? Would you rather take a prescribed menu and follow it? Do you want to join a gym? Would you be better off buying an exercise video and working out at home?

➤ Look for a buddy. You must know at least one other person who wants to lose weight or who just wants to learn how to eat better. Talk about losing weight together. Ideally this will be someone you can talk to, plan with, eat with on occasion, and exercise with on a regular basis. Maybe you can find a food buddy and an exercise buddy.

➤ Start with small, do-able changes. Maybe you have to eat better before you eat less. A small change in your daily routine might be eating a piece of fruit every afternoon in place of your usual candy-bar snack.

NutriTip
If what you've been doing all along to lose weight hasn't been working for you, you have to change something. The more open you are to making lifestyle changes, the easier it will be for you to lose weight.

➤ Be realistic. I can give you all kinds of tips and strategies for getting through the day without overeating, but they won't all work for you. I might say it's okay to have a couple of chocolate chip cookies every day at lunchtime when they're part of an overall healthy eating plan. If you can't keep a box of cookies in the house without eating the whole thing, however, don't buy the box. If you want to be able to eat a cookie every day, you might have to buy them individually at a bakery. You might have to get out of the cookie habit altogether until you're feeling more in control. Think about it. Be realistic about what works for you, or you'll only set yourself up for failure.

First Things First

It's easy to get overwhelmed if you start thinking about everything that's involved in losing weight. So don't. Trying to change and control too many things at once sounds like a recipe for disaster to me. Put your blinders on, and focus on one small change at a time. You're going to ease into this. What's the first thing you need to do? Change your attitude? Change your snacking habits? Change your sneakers?

Maybe the first thing you need to do is make a short list of some of the things you need to do! As with any other "to do" list, prioritize. Don't put buying an expensive piece of exercise equipment first on your list unless you can commit to using it. You might not be ready for such a big move. (If you are, go for it!) Maybe the first thing on your list should be to give away (throw away?) all the junk food in your kitchen. What else? How about moving the candy bowl off your desk at work tomorrow. Next? Maybe reading Chapter 4 of this book. And so on. This is a reminder list—small steps you want to take soon that add up to big changes later. Now. Throw out those chips. Okay, that's enough for today. Done. Check it off your list. Doesn't that feel good?

The Least You Need to Know

➤ Children pick up many of their bad eating habits from their parents and other family members.

➤ There's a genetic link to being overweight, but scientists are still trying to figure out exactly what it means.

➤ The way you eat can affect your mood, just as your mood can affect the way you eat.

➤ Your family and friends might have a hard time adjusting to a "new you." Help them help you.

➤ No matter what your family history is, you can lose weight whenever you're ready.

➤ Setting reasonable goals and making small lifestyle changes are the first steps to losing weight.

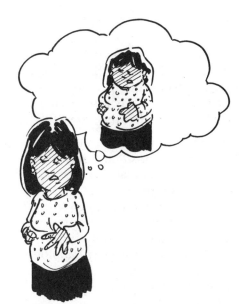

Chapter 4

Heavy Thoughts

In This Chapter

➤ The power of negative thinking

➤ How you can stop feeling guilty about eating

➤ Do you have realistic expectations?

➤ Recognizing the signs of disordered eating

What's on your mind? Food, right? If thinking about food makes you smile, maybe you can skip this chapter. This chapter is for people who feel sad, guilty, afraid, and down-right confused whenever they think about food.

Some overweight people are truly "fat and happy." If you love and accept yourself at any weight, you're one of the very lucky ones. Too many overweight people spend much of their time wishing they were thin. Some take drastic measures, even do dangerous things, to try to be skinnier. Then there are people who aren't overweight at all, but they're miserable because they're obsessed with their bodies and the food they eat, weighing themselves all the time, always putting themselves on diets, and never eating enough food. How can you be happy when you're hungry all the time?

Mind Power

Are you feeling upbeat and positive, ready to get out there and shake up the world? Or are you kicking yourself because you haven't lost any weight this week? If your attitude is "I can do anything, even lose weight," then you know what? You probably will. If your constantly telling yourself "I'll never succeed," then that could just as easily turn out to be true. You'll do whatever your mind tells you to do, even fail. Your mind is that powerful.

Guru's Corner

"Our self-talk is to us like water is to a fish. We don't think about it much because it's always there, surrounding us, a part of what we are. Just as the fish navigates through water, we navigate through life guided by our thoughts. Often we're swimming in negativity. The fish never becomes the water, but we can become the negative thoughts we have about ourselves."

—Lewis Pincus, D.O., founder, To Life! Lifestyle Change Workshops, Dallas, Texas

There's a new name for negative thinking. It's called negative self-talk. It includes all the not-so-nice things you say to yourself throughout the day that make you feel so bad about yourself—such as "I'm so stupid" and "I'm a fat pig." Do you always blame yourself when things go wrong? Do you constantly criticize yourself and call yourself names? That's negative self-talk. You can get into such a habit of negative thinking that you can't see any happiness down the road. You think all the negative stuff is true and will be true forever. The funny thing is that most of what you're telling yourself isn't even true now!

The danger of negative self-talk is that it turns into negative self-opinion. "I can't cook" turns into "I'm no good at anything." "I blew my diet" turns into "I'll never lose weight." Keep thinking that way, and you'll start to believe it! You'll start to see yourself as a failure. When your self-esteem gets that low, you don't think you deserve anything good. You might not think you deserve to be fit and healthy. Please, don't go there!

Dieting can make anyone feel like a failure, especially if you've done it over and over again and haven't been able to keep the extra weight off. You're doomed the minute you go on a diet because most diets are designed to fail. A diet sets you up to lose weight temporarily and then gain it back. How many times can you watch yourself try and fail to lose weight without feeling bad about it? But you didn't fail. The diet failed you. Breaking the habit of negative self-talk helps you stop blaming yourself for failures that aren't yours.

It takes a lot of practice to stop a cycle of negative self-talk because these thoughts become so automatic. You can change the way you think and feel about yourself. The first step is recognizing your negative thoughts. Then you can actively try to change them. Listen to yourself carefully. When you have a negative thought, stop what you're doing. Ask someone close to you to let you know when you're putting yourself down. Then you'll start to hear the negativity yourself. Try to replace the negative thought with something positive. For instance, if you hear yourself say "I look fat," replace it with "I look so young for my age" or "My skin looks great today." If you can't come up with a positive thought, come up with solutions to your negative situation. As soon as you say

"I look fat," follow up with "I can do something about this." Better yet, come up with something specific such as "I'm going to eat more fruit today" or "I'm going to find a personal trainer." Coming up with small immediate solutions can make it easier to feel hopeful about the bigger picture.

Advice from Losers

"Even though I have a husband who loves and supports me, I was always feeling lonely and depressed. No matter what anyone told me, I felt like a failure. These were old, old feelings I'd never been able to shake. Then I just got fed up and decided to start listening to what other people were saying about me, not what I was saying about myself. This past year I've lost 20 pounds, thanks to three simple changes I made in my life. I drink more water and I walk every day, but the big change was in my attitude about myself. Now I get up every morning and tell myself I'm special and worth something. It took a while, but you know what? I believe it!"

—Connie T.

Mind Games

If you're a "list person," it might help to write down your thoughts. Make three columns on a sheet of paper. In the first column, list all those negative feelings and concerns you have about yourself. Get it all out! In the second column, next to each negative item, jot down a possible solution. In the third column, next to each solution, write something positive. If your negative feeling is "I look like a big egg," your solution might be "Join a gym." Your positive thought might be "I can start getting fit right now."

Here's a great little ritual that might help you get rid of negative thoughts and confirm positive ones. I learned this from my friend Wendye, who does it almost every New Year's Eve with her mother as a symbolic way of ringing out the old and bringing in the new. Write down all your negative thoughts on a piece of paper. Read it over and then crumple up the paper or tear it into pieces. Burn it. That's right. Watch all those negative feelings go up in smoke. (Please do this safely and drown your ashes in water before disposing of them!) Now take a nice, small, clean piece of paper. (Small enough to carry in your wallet for inspiration.) Write down some positive feelings and affirmations, some hopes and dreams, even just single words that represent what you want to bring into your life. Don't feel silly. This list is just for you. No one else has to see it. Sometimes when I do this, I just write single words that represent ways I want to be and things I want to have in my life. Words such as calm, love, strength. I know this is the hard part because for many of us, it's so much easier to come up with negative feelings. If you can't think of anything right now, you can borrow from my list:

➤ Self-assurance

➤ Peace of mind

➤ Safety

➤ Choices

➤ Sanity

➤ Energy

➤ Trust

➤ Freedom from stress

These exercises will make you more aware of what's going on in your mind and what might be holding you back from losing weight. They can help you clarify how you feel about yourself and change your habit of negative self-talk into something more positive. Basically, you're changing your entire belief system, and that's not an easy job. A simple list of positive words can be an inspiration. A list of solutions gives you some direction so you can start taking real steps toward that change. You'll be a lot more motivated when you get yourself into a more positive frame of mind.

Picture Perfect

Do you know anyone who's perfect? I don't. Yet we often expect perfection from ourselves, and when we don't live up to those expectations, we start to see ourselves as failures. We compare ourselves to other people who we think are better looking or more successful or skinnier or happier. We're so critical! Very often, the opinions we have of ourselves aren't even based on real facts. We tell ourselves things that aren't even true. The worst part is that we believe it.

No Weigh!
Don't hesitate to seek the help of a professional counselor or psychotherapist who specializes in eating disorders if you're struggling with poor self-esteem or deep feelings of guilt related to food.

We all have this inner critic that lives in our minds somewhere. The critic's sole purpose seems to be to point out all our flaws, every mistake we make, and every way that we don't match up to someone else. I say, kill the critic!

No Guilt, No Blame

Here's why guilt is no good: Guilt is about the past. It's about something that's already happened. Guilt implies you've done something wrong and haven't fixed it. You're carrying around the weight of an unresolved problem. You're working in the present right now, looking toward the future. What good is the guilt you're feeling?

As an overweight person, you've probably come up with a gazillion reasons to feel guilty. Some or all of these guilt-inducers probably sound familiar to you:

➤ Eating more than you should

➤ Eating certain types of food

➤ Not eating food offered by someone else

➤ Bingeing

➤ Not living up to a promise to lose weight

➤ Not keeping weight off

➤ Not losing as much weight as you planned

➤ Feeling like giving up

➤ Eating at night

➤ Throwing up

Guilt, like all negative emotions, gets in the way when you're trying to lose weight. Why? A big part of losing weight and keeping it off is relearning to love and enjoy food. How can you love and enjoy something you feel guilty about?

Whose Guilt Is It, Anyway?

If you feel guilty about food, you probably feel guilty about a lot of other things, too. Are you a perfectionist? If you are, then you must feel guilty about everything because you're never living up to any of your own standards. Give it up! We let guilt sit and gather dust in our heads, but it really isn't necessary. All you have to do is make amends. If you're really guilty of something, admit it and get on with your life! If you've said or done something unkind to someone, apologize. You can always remedy a situation and once you do, there's nothing to feel guilty about anymore. Sometimes we feel guilty on behalf of other people. Maybe your mother or father or spouse did something wrong, and you're carrying the guilt for them. Give it back! It's not your job to shoulder the guilt of the world.

> **Guru's Corner**
> "When you use food to feed emotions, the satisfaction you get is only temporary. To really be satisfied, you have to find other ways to deal with your emotions. You have to learn to feed that special kind of hunger with loving people, positive self-talk, and assertive action, not with food."
>
> —Alice Katz, M.S., psychotherapist and author of *Eating Without Guilt* (Self-Counsel Press, 1991)

> **NutriTip**
> If you overeat for emotional reasons, you have to get to the root of the problem. Try substituting words for food when you're feeling guilty, lonely, or angry. Instead of eating, write your thoughts and feelings down in a journal as soon as you have them and try to analyze your feelings.

Do you apologize for yourself all the time? That's a form of guilt. Do you feel guilty just for existing as an overweight person? Many people do. Guilt suggests that you've done something wrong. What, exactly, did you do? Overeat? Gain weight? So what? Overeating isn't wrong. Neither is gaining weight. Rape is wrong. Child abuse is wrong. Tripping old ladies is wrong. Getting fat might be unpleasant, but it isn't wrong.

Forgive and Forget

You have to let go of guilt, right now. Otherwise you'll just keep punishing yourself for crimes you didn't commit. The pain of guilt is punishment in itself, and you certainly don't deserve that. The anger you must feel about feeling guilty all the time is a form of self-punishment too because it can drive you straight to the refrigerator! (There's more about anger in later chapters.)

Do yourself a big favor. Figure out why you feel guilty. What are you blaming yourself for? Write it down if you can. Examine your guilt. Why is it there? What purpose does it serve? Guilt, like other emotions, always serves a purpose. It could be that by holding on to feelings of guilt, you can't move forward in life. Deep down, you might be happy about that. You don't have to do any work! You don't have to change! Guilt might be the best excuse you have for staying fat. If you let go of your guilt, what will you put in its place? This might not make sense to you at first, but think about it. Change is scary for most people. It's easier to stay where you are than it is to change, and it's pretty amazing how well we manage to stay put.

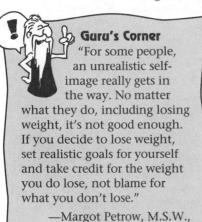

Guru's Corner
"For some people, an unrealistic self-image really gets in the way. No matter what they do, including losing weight, it's not good enough. If you decide to lose weight, set realistic goals for yourself and take credit for the weight you do lose, not blame for what you don't lose."

—Margot Petrow, M.S.W., B.C.D., psychotherapist, New York City

To get rid of guilt and self-blame, you have to forgive yourself, just as you would have to forgive someone else you blame for something. You'll never let go of it until you forgive. I saw a great motto on a bookmark recently that said "When you're angry with someone, you're letting them live in your mind rent-free." Well, that's just as true of guilt and self-blame. You're letting all these negative feelings live in your head and they're not even paying rent! They're not doing anything but taking up space. Kick them out!

Your goal now is to turn guilt into pleasure. The way to do that is break your guilt habit. Remember what I said about negative thinking earlier in this chapter? I discussed substituting positive thoughts for negative. You can do the same thing with the self-talk that makes you feel guilty. How many times have you said to yourself, "I shouldn't eat this," and then gone ahead and eaten it anyway? Then you feel guilty because you did something you told yourself you shouldn't do. Instead, say, "It's dinner time, I'm hungry, and I want to eat something good." You've given yourself permission to eat, so now when you eat, you have nothing to feel guilty about.

What Do You Expect?

What you expect from any diet or exercise program has a lot to do with how much experience you've had trying to lose weight. What you expect will also help determine the outcome. If you don't have much experience, you'll be more open to new weight-loss ideas. Your attitude might be more positive than that of someone who's tried to lose weight over and over again. If you've had your fair share of dieting, you'll probably be more open to ideas that worked for you in the past and less willing to try anything that didn't work before or that you didn't enjoy.

Expectations have a lot to do with how confident you feel about yourself and about any eating plan you develop. If you can give positive answers to the following questions, you probably have confidence in the diet plan you choose (more about this in Part 3, "Small Steps You Can Take Right Now") and will probably get off to a flying start:

> What do you actually think will happen when you start a new eating plan?
>
> Are you ready and willing to change the way you eat?
>
> Can you stick to a new plan?
>
> Does the plan (once you've chosen it) suit your lifestyle?
>
> Will you lose the weight you want to lose in the amount of time you want to lose it?
>
> Why will the new plan "work"?

I want to include a word about unreasonable expectations, such as wanting to lose ten pounds by the end of next week or thinking you can stick to a low-calorie diet plan just because it comes with special nutritional supplements. This is how we get into trouble and set ourselves up to fail. There's no easy way. You're better off starting with lower expectations—a loss of a pound or two a week—so you'll have a better shot at getting there and staying there. Then, if you lose a little more, it'll be a bonus.

NutriTip
The attitude you have about yourself affects your attitude about food. If you trust yourself, you're more likely to trust that your eating habits will improve and that you'll be able to lose weight without depriving yourself and while eating foods you love.

NutriTip
If you're low on confidence, this might not be the time to make big changes in your eating life. Are you trying to change for someone else? Maybe other things happening in your life right now are affecting your sense of self-assurance. If so, ask yourself if you'd be better off solving those problems first.

Eating Disorders

Millions of people suffer from eating disorders. The three most common eating disorders are anorexia, bulimia, and binge eating disorder. Put simply, people with anorexia don't eat enough, people with bulimia overeat and then vomit or use laxatives to purge, and people with binge eating disorder overeat way beyond fullness but usually don't starve or purge themselves. Eating disorders aren't simple at all. They're very complicated and they can be quite serious, evenly deadly.

No Weigh!
Parents who make too big a fuss over what their daughters eat and how much they weigh can unknowingly contribute to eating disorders in young girls. If you're a parent, do not put too much emphasis on your daughter's weight and physical appearance. If you're concerned, ask your pediatrician for advice.

The problem affects mostly young women, but anyone, male or female, can develop an eating disorder at any age. Parents of young athletes should be aware that their children might be under extra pressure to lose weight from coaches and teammates. Young women are particularly vulnerable because they're more likely to go on strict and dangerous diets in an attempt to look more like a favorite model or athlete. Unfortunately, models and athletes themselves often suffer from eating disorders.

Anorexia Nervosa

People with anorexia literally starve themselves. No matter how much they weigh, they think they're too fat and can spend entire days trying to burn off all the calories they eat. People with anorexia

➤ Refuse to eat

➤ Pretend not to be hungry

➤ Lose as much as 15 percent or more of body weight or any large amount of weight in a short period of time

➤ Show an extreme fear of being fat

➤ Exercise excessively

➤ Suffer from constipation

➤ Lose menstrual cycles

➤ Complain of bloating or nausea after eating a normal amount of food

➤ Think they're fat even when they're thin

➤ Binge and purge

Bulimia

People with bulimia binge eat and then purge. They often

➤ Are normal weight or overweight

➤ Feel out of control when eating

➤ Eat secretly

➤ Feel ashamed and depressed after overeating

➤ Eat a large amount of food but don't gain a lot of weight

➤ Disappear after eating (usually into the bathroom to induce vomiting)

➤ Abuse alcohol or drugs

➤ Become dependent on laxatives, diuretics, emetics, or diet pills

➤ Have dental problems caused by stomach acid on their teeth

Binge Eating Disorder

You don't necessarily have binge eating disorder just because you sometimes overeat. People with binge eating problems might also

➤ Eat abnormally large quantities of food in one sitting, such as a half-gallon of ice cream, even when they're not hungry

➤ Feel out of control when eating

➤ Eat more quickly than usual

➤ Eat until uncomfortably full

➤ Eat alone out of embarrassment at the amount of food they're eating

➤ Feel depressed, guilty, or disgusted with themselves after overeating

Guru's Corner

"If you have binge eating disorder, you might also be depressed. You're not alone and you should seek help. First, talk to your physician. If he or she isn't familiar with the disorder, find a licensed psychotherapist who is. Your treatment may include cognitive behavioral therapy combined with an antidepressant such as Paxil, Prozac, or Zoloft, which often helps reduce or eliminate binges."

—Michael D. Myers, M.D., member, Academy of Eating Disorders and the North American Association for the Study of Obesity

The Medical Consequences of Disordered Eating

People with anorexia put themselves at risk of developing a variety of medical conditions, including dehydration, lowered blood pressure, mild anemia, irregular and diminished menstrual periods, brain shrinkage, irregular heart rhythms, and heart failure. People with bulimia often wear down the outer layer of enamel on their teeth from the acid in vomit and suffer from swollen glands and inflamed esophagus. They also increase their risk of heart failure from the loss of essential minerals. Anyone with binge eating disorder is at risk of developing all the medical conditions associated with obesity, such as gallbladder disease, heart disease, and some forms of cancer.

Treating Eating Disorders

Eating disorders are complicated, and sometimes it takes a whole team of experts to treat them properly. The best team includes an internist, a psychotherapist, perhaps a psychopharmacologist (an expert in medications used to treat eating disorders), and a nutritionist who specializes in eating disorders. You might not need to call on all of them at once, but each professional would probably want to confer with any others who have been involved in your case.

NutriTip
If you think someone you know has an eating disorder, approach them in a caring, supportive way. You'll probably get some resistance at first, so get help from family members and friends. Don't give up. The sooner this person gets help, the better chance there is for complete and permanent recovery.

You can save the life of someone with an eating disorder by helping them get treatment. Friends, relatives, teachers, physicians, therapists, and even strangers can all play a role in steering an eating-disorder person toward help. Local hospitals and university medical centers are good places to start. You can find information on the World Wide Web (check out Healthtouch Online at http://www.heathtouch.com/level1/leaflets/102952/102952.htm) and pick up literature from local health organizations and self-help groups. You can also get information from

National Institute of Mental Health
Information Resources and Inquiries Branch
5600 Fishers Lane, Room 7C-02
Rockville, MD 20857
(301) 443-4513

National Eating Disorders Organization (NEDO)
66-55 South Yale Ave.
Tulsa, OK 74136
(918) 481-4044

The Least You Need to Know

➤ When you talk to yourself in a negative way, you start to believe what you say, even when it isn't true.

➤ To break a habit of using negative self-talk, you have to listen to yourself and start replacing negative thoughts with something positive.

➤ Start off with realistic expectations and you won't be disappointed in your diet plan.

➤ If you feel that you might have an eating disorder, ask for a doctor's opinion.

➤ The vast majority of overweight persons do not have a clear eating disorder. For them, the disorder lies in the imbalance between the food they eat and the energy they expand.

Part 2
So Many Ways to Lose

What follows in these next few chapters is sort of a history of diets and dieting methods. You'll probably recognize many of them; perhaps you've tried a few yourself. If you have, then you probably know that most diets don't work. "Oh," you might say, "They worked for a while." I say if they worked, you wouldn't be reading this book right now!

Along with all of the diets that don't work, you'll learn what does work when you're trying to lose or maintain weight. By the end of this part, you'll be able to separate diet fact from diet fiction and start working on a plan that will work for you, once and for all.

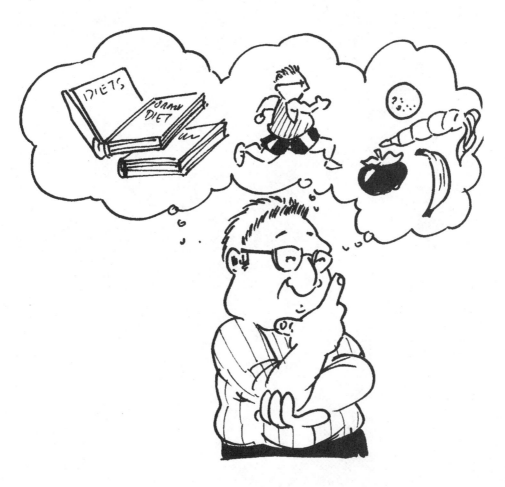

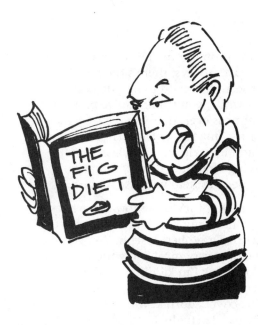

Chapter 5

The Good, the Bad, and the Ugly

In This Chapter

➤ Diets that have come and gone—and a few that have stuck around

➤ Sorting through the confusing messages we get about how to lose weight

➤ How to choose a sensible weight-loss plan

➤ Should you take diet drugs?

➤ What are the alternatives?

Think of all the ways you can lose weight. You can join a diet center. You can go to a private doctor or nutritionist. You can buy a book, a video tape, or a computer program. You can join a gym or buy a treadmill. You can swallow diet pills or have your fat slurped out with a suction machine.

Americans spend more than $30 billion a year trying to lose weight. That's big business. Add to that figure the hundreds of millions spent on obesity research, and you've got quite a hefty sum. There seem to be more failures and disappointments than success stories, and we still don't know how to prevent obesity, so it doesn't look like we're getting our money's worth. This chapter gives an overview of some of the many ways we've tried to lose weight.

Dieting Through the Decades

We're constantly bombarded with magazine ads, book promotions, TV commercials, and infomercials promising easy new ways to slim down fast. Always, there's the promise of a perfect plan that doesn't really exist—promises that seem too good to be true because they are. If something happens to work for you for a while, you think you've finally found the miracle! It's not until you look back, weighty as ever, that you realize your last diet didn't work any better than the one before it or the one before that. That's why it's so important to develop your own personal health and lifestyle plan and learn what really works for you so you won't be duped into buying a product or a plan that can't deliver what it promises or give you what you really need to help you lose weight.

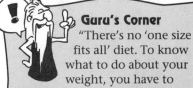

Guru's Corner

"There's no 'one size fits all' diet. To know what to do about your weight, you have to figure out how you got heavy in the first place. Sometimes exercise is your best first step. If you've gained weight simply from overeating, you might be better off focusing on food first."

—Steven Jonas, M.D., coauthor, with Linda Konner, *Just the Weigh You Are* (Chapters Publishing, 1997)

Some diets are so bizarre that they somehow come back around to being sane. One of my personal favorites is the Chocolate Lover's Diet by Dr. Robert Joseph. You get to eat a piece of chocolate before every meal. Now there's a plan I can stick to for life! You think I'm kidding; don't you? Many people snickered and rolled their eyes when this paperback appeared, its cover adorned with a bikini-clad woman and her candy bar. I actually liked it because the basic plan included balanced menus and you got to look forward to eating chocolate at least three times a day. Makes sense to me!

If you've been around for a few years, you've seen some interesting diet ideas come and go. Some of them got more attention than a moon landing. Some stood the test of time and are still around, a few have helped us lose weight, and some should be immediately reported to the diet police if they ever surface again.

Metrical was a hit in the 1960s as the first commercial liquid diet food. Now we call them "meal replacement products."

Also in the '60s, Weight Watchers came out with its first programs, which included support groups and lessons in behavior modification and which were based on "exchanges" of similar-type foods.

One of the first new approaches of the '70s, Dr. Atkins' *Diet Revolution* sold more than 10 million copies and is still going strong, even though most health experts advise us to stay away from this high-protein, very low-carbohydrate plan.

The Grapefruit diet (also called the Mayo diet although it is not associated with or condoned by the Mayo Clinic) had '70s dieters believing that if they ate half a grapefruit before each meal, some magical component of the fruit would help burn off calories from other foods. This diet was high in meat and fat and low in calories and contained no milk or grain foods.

A few other approaches—the Pritikin Plan, Scarsdale diet, Beverly Hills diet, Cambridge diet, Rotation diet, Champagne diet, and Fit for Life diet—emerged in the '80s. The Pritikin Plan, developed by food faddist Nathan Pritikin, encouraged a very low-fat, low-protein, low-calorie diet as a means to curing a variety of ills. When Pritikin's son Robert took over the family business, he loosened the rules a little, letting in a little fun in the form of sugar and alcohol.

Slim-Fast was introduced as a liquid diet formula used to replace one or two normal meals a day.

The Complete Scarsdale Medical Diet promised you could lose 20 pounds in 2 weeks by eating a lot of steak and skipping the bread.

No Weigh!
Avoid any diet that encourages quick weight loss. Losing weight too quickly can cause dehydration, dizziness, and emotional stress, and, in the long run, you get so hungry you'll just end up overeating. Strive to lose about 1 pound a week by making small, gradual changes in your usual eating habits. That's how you develop a lifetime plan you can stick to.

The Beverly Hills Diet allowed nothing but fruit, and only very specific fruit, for the first ten days. This could make you feel very sick to your stomach; then you wouldn't want to eat anyway.

The Cambridge Diet was a high-protein diet-in-a-glass. For weeks, you were supposed to consume nothing but a reconstituted powder three times a day. Yuck!

The Rotation Diet had us rotating our caloric intake to prevent our metabolisms from slowing down. For the first week, women got to eat only 600 to 900 calories a day. The following week, it was 1,200 calories. Then, we returned to the lower number of calories for another week. And so on and so on.

Advice from Losers

"I've always used food to deal with life's ups and downs. I overate whenever I broke up with a boyfriend and whenever I got anxious over taking tests. I overate through two divorces and a hysterectomy. I tried crash diets, group programs, diet doctors, diet pills, and every fad diet. I always regained any weight I lost. Finally I went to a dietitian to learn how to eat properly and find healthy ways to deal with situations that trigger overeating. I love to paint landscapes and I started up again. Now when I have a problem, I know what to do. Instead of eating, I paint."

—Meryl M.

The Champagne Diet rewarded us with a glass of bubbly for suffering through a 1,200 calories a day. Here's to happy weight loss!

The *Fit for Life* diet promises you'll lose weight if you never combine certain foods, such as meat and bread, at the same meal. The theory, which is unusual, to say the least, is that your body can't digest more than one "concentrated" food at a time and that you must eat certain types of foods at certain times of the day. Otherwise, according to the authors, you get fat and toxic because food gets stuck and rots in your body. Oh, yuck!

Now we enter the '90s. *Eat More, Weigh Less* is Dr. Dean Ornish's plan for reducing fat to less than ten percent of your total calories and losing weight on a vegetarian diet. Many experts feel that because of the fat restriction, Ornish's plan is too difficult for the average person to follow.

The Zone brought back the high-protein diet and promised greater energy and physical performance, freedom from hunger, and optimal health. And you could eat fat again! The Zone was touted as "not a diet but a lifelong hormonal control program." Can you say insulin-glucagon axis?

The Cabbage Soup Diet promised, and delivered, quick weight loss for anyone who could follow a plan that included days of eating nothing but cabbage soup and bananas.

The Hacker's diet started serving up some tasty food bytes on the World Wide Web. Why not?

Mixed Messages

A news magazine ran a cover story titled, "Does It Really Matter If You're Fat?" The title sort of implied that it doesn't really matter. Read the article and you find out it does matter. The author wasn't talking about self-acceptance; the subject was health. The gist of the story was that it might be okay healthwise to be overweight if you exercise and stay aerobically fit. In other words, you can be fat and fit at the same time. You also find out that carrying around extra body fat still puts you at higher risk of getting any number of diseases. You learn there's not a lot of new information in that area. I think it's confusing to read such articles. It's a little dangerous for all those people who walk by the newsstand, glance at the cover, and don't buy the magazine or read the article. What those people take away with them is the subtle message they get from the cover line: Maybe it's okay to be fat.

It's no wonder we get confused and just want to hear that it's okay to be fat. There are too many conflicting messages out there about nutrition and weight loss. Don't count calories; count fat grams! No! Calories do count after all! No! Try this high carb plan! No! The way to go is high protein! How can you decide which message to listen to when it's always changing? It's difficult because there are so many gimmicks out there, and the gimmick masters know how to twist the truth here and there to convince you that

No Weigh!
Kids shouldn't be on calorie-restricted diets that were developed for adults because they need to get enough calories for proper growth. If your child needs to lose weight, check with his pediatrician. It might make more sense to encourage him to exercise more and eat better foods rather than eat less food.

they know the best way to weight loss. Remember one thing: You can lose weight once and for all by learning and living some of the basics of good nutrition. When you do that, you become an educated consumer and it gets easier to sort through all the different messages you receive from different books, magazines, television shows, Web sites, and the proverbial grapevine.

Low Fat's Where It's At, or Is It?

Sometime in the mid-1980s, counting grams of fat became the new way to lose weight. The message that went out was that calories don't matter as much as fat. You only get fat from eating fat, I heard people say. I also heard things such as, if you stick to a low-fat diet, you can eat an extra 200 calories a day. I really wanted to believe that one! I had my 50 jelly beans all lined up.

The news about fat also had quite an impact on the food industry. We demanded that food manufacturers develop reduced-fat and fat-free versions of all our fatty favorites.

Boy, did we get them! And boy, did we eat them! We've gained an average of eight pounds per person over the years since the products started coming out. I hate to say it, but it's not the food. It's us. We're always looking for magic bullets. We thought we found one in low-fat fudge, but once again, it was too good to be true.

Don't get me wrong. A reasonably low-fat diet—one that provides 20 to 30 percent of calories from fat—is certainly good for your health. It can be good for your weight, too, as long as you don't overdose on low-fat food products. You can't eat all the potato chips you want just because they're 50 percent lower in fat. You can eat a reasonable amount of chips, just as you always could, as part of an otherwise healthy diet. Yeah, I know. B-o-r-i-n-g!

NutriTip
To lose or maintain weight, you have to watch calories as well as fat and balance the amount of food you eat with exercise. Eat just 100 extra calories a day, the amount in a small banana, an ounce of cream cheese, or two fig bars, and you'll gain ten pounds over the course of a year if you don't increase your activity.

Calories Come, Calories Go

They say that what goes around, comes around. Well, whoever "they" are must know something about dieting. Back in the 1950s, calorie counting was all the rage among women who wanted to lose weight. No one had thought of it before! At least that's what a lot of people believed at the time. (Don't we always think our particular generation is the first to discover anything and everything?) The truth is that calorie counting goes back at least as far as 1918, when Dr. Lulu Hunt Peters defined calories and how to count them in her book, *Diet and Health with Key to the Calories*. Back then, Dr. Peters advised a daily diet that was low in fat and high in carbohydrates and provided 1,200 calories. Sound familiar?

Calories got lost in the shuffle when counting fat grams became a fad. People were chanting "calories don't count!" but now we know better. Calories do count when it comes to losing and maintaining weight. They always did and they always will. You simply can't eat everything in sight just because it's low in fat. Well, you can, of course, but then you can't expect to lose weight or stay the weight you are.

Protein's In, Protein's Out

I knew I was getting old when a client told me that everyone at her gym was losing weight on a high protein diet and she wanted to do the same. My first thought was, "I remember those diets from the '70s, and they're not a good idea." When I expressed this to my client, she stared back blankly. It wasn't what she wanted to hear and she wasn't even born until the '70s. My references and age-old wisdom meant nothing to her, so I stuck with the cold, hard facts.

There's not much bread on a high-protein diet—no bagels, no muffins, no French toast. (That would end it for me right there!) High-protein diets are usually low in carbohydrates. As soon as you cut back on carbohydrates in your diet, you lose water weight. That's why people who go on a high-protein diet feel quick results. So what's the problem?

> **NutriTip**
> Well-balanced meals that contain mostly carbohydrates from vegetables and starches, some protein from meat, dairy, or beans, plus a little fat are best for losing weight and maximizing energy in the long run. Balanced meals, spaced no more than four or five hours apart, keep your blood sugar even and your appetite under control. You'll have longer-lasting energy and stay satisfied longer.

Your brain needs a sugar called glucose for energy. No other fuel will do. Glucose comes from carbohydrates, and if you don't eat enough of them, your brain could be in trouble. What happens instead is that your muscles break down to provide certain types of protein that your body can use to make glucose. That way, at least your brain gets fed. Meanwhile, as your body starts using fat stores for energy, you develop a condition known as ketosis, which indicates that you're not eating enough food, especially carbohydrates. Next your metabolism slows down and you stop burning fat. At this point, your body, and your health, are totally whacked out. It's similar to what happens if you fast for any length of time. You might lose your appetite and lose some weight, but you're losing your health at the same time.

Up with Carbs, Down with Carbs

I distinctly remember a newspaper headline that said "Pasta makes you fat!" Pasta doesn't make you fat, but some dubious research led some ordinary people to believe that the reason they're fat is because they can't correctly metabolize certain types of carbohydrates such as those found in pasta and bread. These "carbohydrate addicts" also believed that eating carbs triggered cravings for more carbs. The only solution they could propose was eating fewer carbohydrates.

At the same time that carbohydrates were criticized, however, high carbohydrate diets were "in." Talk about food confusion! It's always been true, and it remains true, that most of your calories should come from carbs. That's carbs of all kinds, of course: fruits, vegetables, rice, cereal, bread, and pasta—not to mention an occasional cookie. On a varied, balanced diet, you can eat any type of carbohydrate you want and still lose weight. Just remember what I just said about calories!

Who's Telling the Truth?

The best person to rely on, always, is yourself! How many times have you put your faith and fate in the hands of others, only to be disappointed? How often do you roll your eyes, now, thinking "Oh, no, not another diet." Even if you do follow a fad diet for a while, you probably know deep down that something's fishy. It isn't going to "work." As long as you're not hurting yourself, it can be fun to try different eating plans for a day or two. (I admit it; I once ate only cabbage soup and bananas for a day.) It can keep you aware of what's going on in weight-loss land and teach you lessons, both good and bad, for the future. Just don't delude yourself into thinking that this next new diet fad is "the one" that will make you lean and mean. Mean, maybe, if you're not eating enough food, but not lean. Not in the long run.

> **NutriTip**
> The best weight-control advice comes from doctors, dietitians, and exercise physiologists who are trained in the field, and, if necessary, psychotherapists who specialize in eating disorders. Good advice doesn't always have to come directly from a health professional. It can come second-hand from a knowledgeable person, but think twice about anyone who's selling anything more than sound advice and counsel.

It's usually best to seek help from experts. They're easy to find. They go on television, they write books, they visit Web sites, and they produce videos. When you consider buying a book or videotape about weight control or taking advice from anyone, check the credentials of the authors and experts involved. Is the writer a doctor, a dietitian, an exercise physiologist, or a psychologist? No true professional goes beyond his or her scope of practice without calling in or referring you to other experts. Your personal trainer should only give you limited, basic information about nutrition and weight loss. Most likely, a dietitian won't be an expert on weight training. It's rare that one person can tell you everything you need to know about how to lose weight.

Health-care professionals don't work in health food stores. When I go into health food stores, I often hear the employees giving health advice and promoting "natural" weight-loss products and supplements. Remember that they have to sell products from the store to earn a living. If you wander in looking for weight-loss aids, make sure you know what you're buying. It might be harmless, but it might not come with good advice.

Evaluating Diets and Weight-Loss Plans

The idea that obesity is a disease is somewhat controversial, but many experts agree that it's a chronic condition. The problem is that we often treat it as a brief illness. We pick a diet, go on it, and get off it when we see results or just can't stand it anymore.

The way to lose weight and keep it off is to pick a plan and stick to it. That's more likely to happen if you pick a sensible plan. It doesn't matter whether your weight-loss plan comes from a book, a magazine, a nutritionist, or a commercial diet program. It has to be sensible and it has to fit into your lifestyle. The National Institute of Health recommends you look for these features in any weight-loss or weight-maintenance plan you choose:

No Weigh!
Beware of any diet that eliminates any of the major food groups or singles out any particular type of food as "bad." A weight-loss diet should allow a wide variety of foods so that you not only get all the nutrients you need while eating fewer calories, but you also have a little fun doing it.

NutriTip
For information on the Recommended Dietary Allowances, contact

Food and Nutrition Information Center (FNIC) Room 304 National Agricultural Library, ARS, USDA 10301 Baltimore Ave. Beltsville, MD 20705-2351

You can also get copies of the RDAs from FNIC's Web site:

www.nal.usda.gov/fnic/ Dietary/rda.html

➤ The diet should be safe and should include all the Recommended Daily Allowances (RDAs) for vitamins, minerals, and protein from food. It's virtually impossible to do that on any diet with fewer than 1,200 calories.

➤ The program should be aimed at slow, steady weight loss unless you are in a medically supervised program, and your doctor feels you can safely benefit from faster weight loss. You should expect to lose only about a pound a week during the first week or two. (Initially, you might lose more weight, but much of this loss will be fluids.) The plan should encourage you to set reasonable goals.

➤ Your program should include plans for weight maintenance after you lose weight. Weight maintenance is the most difficult part of controlling your weight, and many plans don't take this into consideration. The program you select should help you permanently change any eating and exercise habits and lifestyle patterns that may have contributed to your weight gain in the past.

➤ The program should provide behavior-modification help. It should include education in healthy eating habits and long-term plans to deal with weight problems. The program should help you incorporate an individually tailored exercise program into your plan.

➤ A commercial weight-loss program should provide you with a detailed statement of fees and costs of additional items such as dietary supplements.

If you plan to lose more than 15 to 20 pounds, have any health problems, or take any medication on a regular basis, see your physician for a checkup before you begin any weight-loss program. If you plan to use a very low-calorie liquid formula diet that provides fewer than 800 calories, you absolutely must be examined and monitored by a medical doctor.

Popping Pills

Plenty of pills—both prescription and over-the-counter—can help you get through the day without overeating. Diet pills, including those you can buy in the drugstore without a prescription, can have serious side effects, such as increased blood pressure, irregular heartbeat, and even liver damage. Some new and popular prescription pills, such as "fen-phen," can cause damage to your lungs. All diet drugs are short-term solutions to weight loss. Ask yourself, and your physician, if the benefits outweigh the risks.

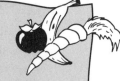

NutriTip
The best weight-loss plans encourage you to

➤ Set realistic goals

➤ Follow a familiar and comfortable meal plan

➤ Eat foods that are readily available in stores where you live

➤ Eat a wide variety of foods from all the major food groups

➤ Exercise on a regular basis

Over-the-Counter Diet Pills

Your local drugstore probably has a whole small section devoted to weight-loss aids and non-prescription diet pills. The active ingredient in many of these pills is an appetite suppressant called phenylpropanolamine (PPA). PPA will curb your hunger pangs, at least for a day or two, but it might also upset your stomach, make you feel dizzy, and increase blood pressure. This is a drug that comes with a long list of reasons why you might not want to take it, such as pre-existing medical conditions and conflicts with other medications. Read the label carefully before you buy.

No Weigh!
Don't be tempted to take laxatives because you think they'll help you lose weight. They won't. You'll still absorb calories. What you might lose if you take laxatives are essential body fluids, and that can lead to serious health problems.

You might be lured into the health food store by signs promising "natural" solutions for weight loss. Many herbal diet pills contain diuretics that cause you to eliminate more water and possibly lose temporary water weight. You won't lose any actual weight with a diuretic. Some weight-loss aids contain drug-like substances that can cause serious side effects such as heart irregularities. Let me also make one thing clear: No grapefruit pill or nutritional supplement that I'm aware of "melts" or "burns" fat. Don't waste your money on any nutritional supplements that make these kinds of weight-loss claims.

Prescriptions for Weight Loss

Some physicians think obesity is a chronic medical condition that is amenable to treatment with prescription medication. Most diet drugs traditionally prescribed by physicians are appetite suppressants used only for short-term treatment, that is, two to three months. A newer generation of drugs is being developed for longer-term use. For someone who is truly obese and who has tried and failed over and over again to lose weight, some physicians feel medication is the best short-term solution.

Diet drugs seem to be most effective during the first six months of treatment. After that, you're likely to maintain your weight or gain some of it back, even though you're still popping pills. If you're thinking about taking prescription diet drugs, keep in mind that when the medication is discontinued, many people gain back the weight they've lost.

Whether or not you should take diet drugs is up to you and your doctor. If your weight is really high and your ability to lose weight is really low, you might be a good candidate for short-term prescription drug therapy. Remember that all drugs have side effects, some more serious than others. Your doctor can help you decide if the health risks associated with being overweight in your particular case outweigh the risks of taking medication.

Alternative Thinking

There are many paths to achieving a healthy body, and when you're struggling with weight, it's helpful to have an open mind. Some alternative approaches, such as ear stapling and hypnosis, haven't lived up to their dubious reputations as aids to long-term weight loss. Others, such as meditation and an occasional day of semi-fasting that includes some solid food, can be helpful tools if you're trying to eliminate stress and break old habits that contribute to overeating.

What's Your Mantra?

Meditation can be a useful way of dealing with stress because it helps quiet all the conflicting thoughts that are causing chaos in your mind. Scientific studies have actually proven that meditation lowers blood pressure. How can it possibly help you lose weight? By reducing stress, you might be able to cut back on overeating and other unhealthy habits. In his book *Eat More, Weigh Less* (Harper Collins, 1993), Dr. Dean Ornish points out that meditation helps you become more aware of the food you eat and how it affects you. If you're paying attention, you'll know when you've had enough and you won't be as likely to overeat.

Fasting

A day without eating? I can hardly imagine it. In some countries, that's called starvation. Fasting is sometimes promoted as a way to "cleanse" your body of pollutants and other toxins that have accumulated over time. Most health experts agree that our bodies don't need special cleaning.

Here's what happens when you don't eat: Your body uses whatever sugar is in your blood for energy. After several hours, when there's no more blood sugar, you start to break down the carbohydrates known as glycogen stored in your muscles and maybe some body fat. When fat is used as the primary source of energy, you form chemical compounds known as ketone bodies. If too many ketones are formed, they can accumulate in your body. You'll become dehydrated and feel ill. It's not a pretty sight. Like any other short-term method, fasting won't help you lose weight because as soon as you stop fasting, you'll gain back any water weight you did lose.

No Weigh!
Any dieting method that causes a drop in your blood sugar or blood pressure is especially risky for anyone with medical problems. If you have health problems such as diabetes, heart disease, or hypertension, you shouldn't go on any type of fast for even a day.

The Least You Need to Know

➤ Stay away from diets that promise quick results or sound too good to be true.

➤ Balance is key to any successful weight-control program. A balanced weight loss plan contains both a moderate decrease in calories and a moderate increase in exercise.

➤ The best weight control plans help you set realistic goals and develop an individual plan for reaching them that includes a wide variety of foods and regular exercise.

➤ Medication of any kind is only a short-term solution for weight loss. Any lost weight might return once you stop taking medication.

➤ Some alternative approaches, such as meditation, might help reduce some of the stress that causes you to overeat.

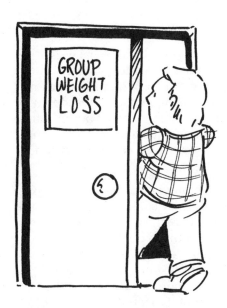

Chapter 6

The Scoop on Group Weight-Loss Programs

In This Chapter

➤ Who's running the weight-loss show?

➤ Medically supervised modified fasting programs

➤ Looking for support?

➤ How to figure out if a group program will work for you

In 1990, the government began investigating advertising claims made by 16 commercial weight-loss systems. All the companies investigated were later charged with misleading the public about the safety, effectiveness, maintenance, or cost of their programs. And you think you're a failure at weight loss!

More than seven million people enroll in commercial weight-loss programs each year, and it's a good guess that most of them expect to lose weight and keep it off. The diet industry as a whole has been much maligned for not living up to its promises of successful weight loss and in many cases, rightly so. Some of the leading group programs have changed their approaches in an attempt not only to save their own butts but to help shrink ours with more up-to-date weight loss plans.

This chapter looks at the most popular group programs so you can evaluate whether one of them might be a useful part of your weight-loss plan.

Commercial Weight-Loss Programs

Program bashers will tell you it's a waste of time and money to join a commercial weight-loss center. They'll say you're just as likely to lose weight on your own. Most statistics show that they're right. For some people, however, that's like saying, "You can quit smoking on your own" or "You can learn how to use a computer without taking a class." It just doesn't make sense for everyone. If you're highly inspired and have the time to teach yourself what you need to know, sure, you can learn anything. If you're not motivated to go it alone and you want support, a group weight-loss program might be for you. Some people actually do lose weight and keep it off with the help of a commercial program.

NutriTip
Counselors who work at commercial weight-loss centers don't necessarily have any formal training in health, nutrition, psychology, or exercise physiology. You might want to seek the additional help of experts outside the program you choose to join.

No Weigh!
You can't live on prepackaged diet food forever. If you join a program that has its own food plan, be sure that part of the plan is to teach you how to prepare healthful meals on your own, with foods you can buy in the supermarket.

There's no way to know which program is best for you until you compare a few. Some people try a number of different programs before settling on one. Besides the well-known national programs, you might want to check out smaller, local programs offered through YMCAs, YWCAs, local community centers, and hospitals. Shop around, and before you commit to any weight-loss plan, be sure to read the section "How to Evaluate a Group Program" at the end of this chapter.

At the very least, a good weight-loss program should include a nutritionally balanced diet combined with exercise recommendations and behavioral counseling. Eating plans vary somewhat from program to program. Some programs include prepackaged food plans, which might appeal to you if you don't want to make any food decisions on your own. Remember that you're making a commitment to eating a lot of convenience foods for a long period of time. If you're used to eating convenience foods, it won't be as difficult as if you were used to eating more fresh foods. Be prepared to pay top dollar for these foods in addition to the program's initial membership fee. Be sure the program also includes a transition plan to teach you how to prepare healthful food on your own. To lose weight in the long run, you have to learn how to make healthier food choices outside the program.

When you spend your hard-earned money on something, you want it to work. If you're spending your money on a diet dream, you want the dream to come true. However, you can't turn the responsibility for your weight completely over to someone or something else without taking some responsibility. Weight-loss programs sell tools as well as promises and many of these tools are worthwhile if you learn how to use them correctly. Become an educated consumer and learn about the realities of weight control so you can feel confident in your choice of program. A group program can provide

➤ **Structure.** Each program has its own approach and its own set of rules to guide you.

➤ **Counseling.** You have someone to talk to and someone to guide you through the program.

➤ **Motivation.** When counseling is included in the program, someone besides yourself is paying attention to your diet and helping to motivate you.

➤ **Support.** Most of the larger programs include group meetings and there's a good chance you'll make new friends and find support among the other members. You'll have an opportunity to learn from other "losers."

If you're pregnant, have a medical condition such as diabetes, kidney disease, or heart disease, take certain medications, or have a history of eating disorders, you might not be accepted into a commercial weight-loss program or you might need written approval from your doctor. Otherwise, most programs accept anyone who has at least ten pounds to lose.

Weight Watchers

Weight Watchers International was the original group weight-loss program, founded in 1963 by Jean Nidetch. Jean was an overweight housewife in Queens, New York, who was concerned about her obsession with cookies. She began by gathering friends in her living room for mutual weight-loss support.

Recognizing that any stress only sabotages our best diet intentions, the powers-that-be at Weight Watchers recently updated the program so that it's a lot less stressful to its members. There's no more weighing of food and a lot less measuring. Bigger portion sizes, more "free" foods, and more indulgences are allowed. With fewer restrictions, the program has become easier to follow. When you follow the Weight Watchers plan, you can choose to trade off more activity for more food. In other words, the more you move, the more you can eat.

Advice from Losers

"I've been overweight my whole life, and I guess I got it from my mother's side of the family. I grew up eating double helpings of everything—two hamburgers instead of one, half a plateful of potatoes instead of half a cup—and never realized I was eating too much food. I never even heard the words "portion control" until I joined Weight Watchers. I want to lose at least 140 pounds. I'm always able to lose the first 40 pounds; then I hit a plateau and I stop losing, give up, and gain the weight back. I wanted to give up this time, too, but my group leader kept working with me. I believed her when she said the plateau would eventually end and I bought the prepayment plan this time so I would stick with it. Finally, after four long months, I'm losing again. You have to have faith!"

—Patty D.

Regular, weekly attendance at group meetings is encouraged. All group leaders are Weight Watchers members who have lost weight on the program and since completed a leader training program. Although cookbooks, videos, and other Weight Watchers products are offered for sale, they're not required to follow the program. Weight Watchers has traditionally been the least expensive of all the commercial weight-loss programs, in great part because you can buy your own food outside of the program.

Jenny Craig

The Jenny Craig weight-management program was founded in Australia in 1983 and introduced in the United States in 1985 by none other than Jenny Craig herself, along with her husband.

No Weigh!
Don't sign up for any weight-loss plan unless you're perfectly comfortable with the program's methods, the cost, and the qualifications of everyone you meet who's involved with the program.

Initially, members must purchase and eat Jenny-Craig–brand, packaged, preportioned foods every day, along with fresh fruits, vegetables, breads, and dairy products. The preplanned menus designed to include Jenny Craig foods are designed to allow you to lose one to two pounds a week. Once you're halfway to your weight goal, you reduce the amount of Jenny Craig foods on your plan and learn more about making your own low-fat foods. In addition to the food products, the Jenny Craig plan includes its own brand of vitamin and mineral supplements.

If you go with the total Jenny Craig program, you'll also do a lot of work on your own, using lifestyle guidebooks and audio fitness tapes that are part of the program. You'll meet once a week with a consultant who helps personalize these materials for you and provides some motivation. There's a special program for teenagers at Jenny Craig, and in 1996, the company began testing a physician-supervised program that includes weight-loss medications for qualified members.

Nutri-System

After helping his own mother lose weight, Philadelphia businessman Harold Katz founded Nutri-System in 1971. Now there are about 2,000 centers, many of which are franchised throughout the United States, Canada, Australia, England, and France. Members buy and use Nutri-System–brand foods and supplement them with some fresh fruits, vegetables, and dairy products.

Counselors at Nutri-System help you figure out how much weight you can expect to lose in an established amount of time and then introduce you to a program they feel will help you do that. In addition to weekly one-on-one counseling sessions, weekly group meetings discuss the basics of food exchanges and portion-controlled eating.

Diet Center

The Diet Center was founded by frustrated dieter Sybil Ferguson in 1970 and has grown to more than 2,000 centers throughout the world. Like Nutri-System and Jenny Craig, the Diet Center program incorporates its own line of products including portion- and calorie-controlled meals, snacks, and drinks, motivational tools such as activity books, and audio cassette fitness and relaxation tapes. Diet Center consultants use a computerized assessment program to pinpoint your individual habits, emotions, eating triggers, and motivation level and help you develop a personal plan.

Advice from Losers

"My group is a permanent part of my lifestyle. But you can't torture yourself or let the rules of a program rule your life. At first, I got into a vicious cycle of starving myself just before weigh-ins and then overeating as soon as it was over. Then I'd be fighting my hunger all week to lose the weight again before the next weigh-in. It took a long time, but now I'm not so hard on myself. I went on a dinner cruise the night before weigh-in last week. In the past, I would've tortured myself and not let myself eat. This time I said, 'Who cares. I'm going to have fun.' And I weighed-in fine."

—Ann Marie L.

Repeat Performances

I've spoken to men and women who've joined and rejoined commercial weight-loss centers no less than half a dozen times. Why do they keep going back? For one thing, they don't want to give up on themselves. Some say they lack willpower on their own. Others tell me they need the structure of an organized program.

It takes the average smoker six or seven tries before he gives cigarettes up for good. Don't feel bad if you've tried to lose weight at least that many times. As a friend of mine once said, "Life keeps teaching you the same lessons over and over again until you get it right." There's a lot to learn when it comes to losing weight. The more you learn, the closer and easier it will be to get to your healthiest weight.

Life in the Fast Lane

If you're at least 20 to 30 percent above your ideal body weight or your BMI is greater than 30, your doctor might recommend a very-low-calorie-diet program offered through a local hospital or medical center. Sometimes these diets are called modified fasts. Under the doctor's care, your diet will consist only of a liquid formula that provides 800 calories or less each day. You won't have to make a single decision about food because, in most cases, you won't be eating any. If you can live this way, you'll lose about 3 to 5 pounds a week and average about 44 pounds over 12 weeks.

A supervised modified fast is the only near-safe way to lose this much weight this quickly. But it's risky. True, it can be helpful if you're very overweight and frustrated by safer, saner plans that move so slowly. If you're a compulsive overeater, this type of diet might help you break bad eating habits and feel more motivated to start losing weight in a more traditional way. Unfortunately, very-low-calorie diets are hazardous to your health. Your body thinks it's being starved and immediately takes measures to protect itself. There aren't enough calories for your body to function normally. Your metabolism might slow, and you might feel sick at times. You actually risk sudden death, although it's very rare. That's why you can only stay on a very-low-calorie diet for a very short period of time and only under the close supervision of a doctor.

No Weigh!
Don't even think about going on a very-low-calorie modified fast diet without medical supervision. These are dangerous diets that can make you very sick if you're not under a doctor's care.

It's also important to know that modified fasts don't work any better than any other type of diet in the long-run and they can be expensive. Weight loss on these programs is dramatic, for sure, but it's short term. Losing weight is easy if you follow this type of program for a couple of months. But keeping the weight off is just as hard or harder as if you lost it slowly. If you sign up for a modified fast, be sure the program includes maintenance. If you don't commit to permanent lifestyle changes that include more physical activity and healthier eating, your weight will quickly come back. Some hospitals have their own, similar modified fasting plans, but the most well-known programs are Medifast, Health Management Resources, and Optifast:

➤ Medifast is a four-phase program that includes a medical evaluation, weight-reduction phase, refeeding phase, and maintenance phase. During the weight reduction phase, women are placed on a 450-calorie liquid diet and men on a 480-calorie liquid diet.

➤ Health Management Resources offers the choice of a very-low-calorie (520 to 800 calories) or a moderately low calorie (800 to 1,000 calories) diet plan that uses a liquid formula or the program's own frozen foods that contain approximately 150 to 230 calories.

➤ Optifast uses an 800-calorie liquid diet formula. To be eligible for this program, you must be at least 30 percent over your ideal body weight. You can enter the program at 20 percent or 60 pounds over if you are at risk of medical problems due to your weight.

Just for Support

Non-profit weight-loss support groups offer motivation and friendship to people who struggle with their weight. These groups don't endorse or promote any particular diet or exercise plans, but they do encourage sensible weight-control practices. They're intended to be safe places where overweight people can feel free to discuss their feelings and find help and encouragement. Meetings are often held in community centers and churches.

Overeaters Anonymous

Like Alcoholics Anonymous and Narcotics Anonymous, Overeaters Anonymous (OA) is a 12-step recovery program. The program provides support for people who are recovering from compulsive overeating and encourages participation in all safe, sensible weight-loss programs. Compulsive overeating is treated as a progressive disease that can be arrested. The foundation of OA is abstinence from overeating, one day at a time, and recovery on physical, emotional, and spiritual levels. Members are encouraged to carry their message of recovery to compulsive overeaters. Anyone who's looking for freedom from food obsession is welcome to get with the program. There are no membership dues or fees, but group members usually make voluntary contributions at meetings to help cover expenses. To find an OA meeting in the United States, Canada, or one of 50 other countries worldwide, look up Overeaters Anonymous in the local business or residential white pages or call (505) 891-2664.

Guru's Corner
"If you hide food or eat in secret, if you can't stop eating when you want to, and if your eating interferes with your relationships, you might have a food addiction. But food isn't the primary problem and recovery doesn't focus on weight loss. You can find help in private psychotherapy and in group self-help programs."

—Kay Sheppard, LMHC, CEDS author of *Food Addiction: The Body Knows* (Health Communications, Inc.)

Take Off Pounds Sensibly (TOPS)

In addition to providing emotional support to its 300,000 members, TOPS provides financial support to obesity researchers. Members of TOPS are encouraged to consult with a physician for weight-loss advice and supervision. In addition to weekly local meetings, members attend group rallies and get-away retreats. At the weekly meetings, members weigh-in privately and then attend a group program designed to help them reach their individual weight-loss goals. The programs include contests, handouts, recipes, and talks given by local health professionals. Members who are so inclined share weight-loss stories during meetings. An inspirational monthly magazine is included in the annual $20 (U.S.) membership fee. To locate a chapter near you, call (800) 932-8677.

How to Evaluate a Group Program

The best way to figure out whether a program is for you is to collect and compare information on different programs in your area. Before you sign up for any group weight-loss program, ask these questions and be sure you're satisfied with the answers:

NutriTip
Check to see if your local hospital, medical center, or university hospital has a weight-management program. Unlike most other commercial programs, medical programs are usually staffed by a team of doctors, dietitians, psychologists, and exercise physiologists. The only drawback is that unless they're covered by your medical insurance, these programs can be expensive.

No Weigh!
Beware of any weight-management program that encourages a loss of more than one to two pounds a week after the first week. If you lose more rapidly than that, you could end up with serious health problems.

➤ How long has the program been around?

➤ What's the total cost of the program, including any special food, supplements, or other products?

➤ What type of professionals—doctors, dietitians, nurses, and counselors—provide their services to members?

➤ How often will you attend meetings or counseling sessions?

➤ Is the program goal-oriented? Will you get help setting positive lifestyle change goals as well as weight-loss goals?

➤ How much weight can you expect to lose each week, and how long will it take for you to reach your goal weight?

➤ How will your weight loss be monitored?

➤ If you're over 35, does the program address your age group?

➤ Does the program include any kind of physical activity recommendations?

➤ Does the program address any special medical needs you might have, such as diabetes or a medical problem that prevents physical activity?

➤ Is a weight-maintenance plan included in the cost of the program? If so, what does the plan provide?

The Least You Need to Know

➤ There are a number of group weight-loss programs you can join if you don't want to lose weight on your own.

➤ Medically supervised, very-low-calorie liquid diet programs are designed for people who are at least 20 or 30 percent above ideal body weight.

➤ If you're simply looking for support, you can join a non-profit group such as Take Off Pounds Sensibly (TOPS) or Overeaters Anonymous (OA).

➤ Compare and evaluate several programs in your area to see what's right for you before you make a financial commitment.

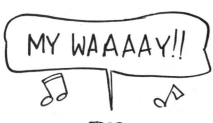

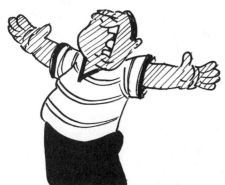

Chapter 7

For Do-It-Yourselfers

In This Chapter

➤ Are you ready to lose weight?

➤ How to assess yourself

➤ Figuring out a plan

➤ Developing a support system

Sometimes people act a lot like their own fat cells. They're not really motivated to give up their fat, especially on their own. They're not ready to start making the lifestyle changes necessary to get fit. But that's not you. You're ready now!

This chapter tells you what it takes to lose weight on your own and helps you assess your own readiness to knock it off once and for all. You'll learn how to provide your own structure, find motivation and support, develop a plan, and monitor yourself. You'll see that it's a whole lot easier than it sounds!

Are You Ready?

You're psyched. You're motivated. You're ready to lose weight. You don't need any help at all, right? Wrong! Even the most independent souls need guidance sometimes. That's why you're reading this book!

What's Your Motivation?

You must be enormously self-motivated if you're willing to take on the challenge of losing weight all by yourself. Do you know where that motivation comes from? Different things motivate different people. One of the best motivators is good health. If you believe that losing weight is a healthy thing to do, it'll be easier to run that last lap or turn down that second helping of pie. At the same time, you must believe that a healthy diet and exercise plan is "worth it." In your mind, it has to be worth the effort it takes to develop a plan and stick to it. You might also be motivated by the pure sense of accomplishment that comes with losing weight and getting fit. It usually feels good to get what you want.

Advice from Losers

"I had just had my baby and wanted to get back in shape but hadn't gotten around to doing anything about it yet. I knew my backside was huge, but since I couldn't really see it, and my husband never said a word, I was sort of ignoring it. It was summer, and I was walking the baby in his carriage when a bicycle messenger pulled up right behind me. He actually said, 'Hey Mama, you had that little baby and your butt sure got big from it!' Talk about motivation! I joined a gym that afternoon and within 6 weeks lost 20 pounds. Sometimes it takes a stranger to tell you the truth!"

—Linda F.

Some motivations for losing weight aren't so good because they don't come from within yourself. You can't successfully lose weight to please someone else. It has to be for you—not for a spouse or a parent or a child or a counselor. Others can *help* motivate you by giving you a lot of support and nudging you in the right direction. For example, it's more than okay to follow the advice of a doctor who suggests you lose weight, but you probably won't be able to lose it if you're not also motivated from within. No one else can be your primary reason for losing weight.

Ready or Not

There's no question that to succeed at weight loss, you need the right attitude. Do you have it? Take the Weight Loss Attitude Quiz from the American Dietetic Association to see if you're ready to commit right now. Circle each answer true or false. (Do not read further before taking the quiz, or you might be tempted to "cheat" a little.)

Weight Loss Attitude Quiz

Circle T for True or F for False.

T F **1.** I've thought a lot about my eating habits and physical activities to pinpoint what I need to change.

T F **2.** I've accepted the idea that I need to make permanent, not temporary, changes in my eating and activities to be successful.

T F **3.** I will only feel successful if I lose a lot of weight.

T F **4.** I accept the idea that it's best if I lose weight slowly.

T F **5.** I'm thinking of losing weight now because I really want to, not because someone else thinks I should.

T F **6.** I think losing weight will solve other problems in my life.

T F **7.** I'm willing and able to increase my regular physical activity.

T F **8.** I can lose weight successfully if I have no "slip-ups."

T F **9.** I'm ready to commit some time and effort each week to organizing and planning my food and activity programs.

T F **10.** Once I lose some initial weight, I usually lose the motivation to keep going until I reach my goal.

T F **11.** I want to start a weight-loss program even though my life is unusually stressful right now.

To score the Weight Loss Attitude Quiz, look at your answers next to items 1, 2, 4, 5, 7, and 9. Score 1 if you answered true and 0 if you answered false. For items 3, 6, 8, 10, and 11, score 0 for each true answer and 1 for each false answer. Now add up the scores of all questions. There's no right score, but the higher your total score, the better your chances of success right now. If you scored 8 or higher, you probably have good reasons for wanting to lose weight now and a good understanding of what you need to do to succeed. If you scored 5 to 7, you might need to reexamine your reasons for losing weight and the methods you would use to do so. If you scored 4 or less, this might not be the right time for you to lose weight because your answers suggest that you might not be able to stick to your plan and lose all the weight you want or to keep off the weight you do lose. No matter what you scored, it might help to read these interpretations for any quiz item where you scored 0.

No Weigh!
There's no reason to hurry when you're trying to lose weight. The more slowly you peel off those extra pounds, the more likely you are to keep them off. Don't forget: You're not just making a commitment to lose weight, you're making a commitment to lifestyle changes that are going to help you lose weight and keep it off for good.

1. It's been said that you can't change what you don't understand. You might benefit from keeping records for a week or longer to help pinpoint when, what, why, and how much you eat and why you can't exercise more often. (See Chapter 9, "Dear Diary....")

2. Making drastic or highly restrictive changes in your eating habits might allow you to lose weight in the short run, but these changes might be too hard to live with in the long run. The same goes for exercise. Both your food and activity plans should be healthful and enjoyable.

3. Most people have fantasies of reaching a weight that's much lower than they can realistically maintain. You might want to rethink your meaning of "success." A successful, realistic weight-loss plan is one that you can comfortably maintain. Take your body type into consideration, and then set small, achievable goals. Your first goal could be to lose a small amount of weight while you learn better eating and exercise habits that will help you maintain the loss.

4. If you think success equals fast weight loss, it will be hard for you to maintain your weight. "Quick-fix" attitudes usually backfire. It's better to lose weight slowly while you learn how to keep the weight off permanently.

5. The desire for and commitment to weight loss must come from you. To lose and maintain weight successfully, you have to take responsibility for your own desires and decide the best way to achieve them. Friends and family are important sources of support, but they can't be your motivation.

6. If you lose weight, you might feel more self-confident and empowered, and the skills you develop to deal with your weight can be applied to other areas of your life. However, anticipating that all your problems will be solved by losing weight is unrealistic and can set you up for huge disappointments.

7. People who get regular, moderate exercise are usually more successful at maintaining their weight. Get moving!

8. Perfection at weight loss is unrealistic. Rather than expect it and see your lapses as catastrophes, look at them as good opportunities to identify problem triggers and come up with new strategies for the future.

9. Successful weight loss requires planning and takes time. You have to be able to make the commitment.

10. Don't ignore any concerns you have about "going the distance" because they might indicate a future problem. Think about why your past efforts at weight loss failed. Work on motivational strategies to get you over these hurdles. Take your effort one day at a time; it's normal to reach a plateau and stay there for a while when you're trying to lose weight.

11. Weight loss itself is a source of stress, so if you're already under stress for other reasons, it might be hard for you to lose weight right now. Try to resolve the other stresses in your life before you begin a weight-loss program.

If you scored high on the readiness quiz, go for it! Do it now! Jump right in! I don't want to sound too effusive, but this is a great time for you to start managing your weight. You're ready to move on to the next section and start taking those baby steps. If you scored medium, you can still jump in and begin your self-assessment exercises, covered in the next section. At the same time, however, go over the quiz answer explanations and see what additional steps you need to take to make sure your weight-loss plan is a success.

Assess Yourself

When you choose to go it alone, you have plenty of flexibility and certainly a lot of personalized attention because you give it to yourself. You also have to do more thinking for yourself. You have to set yourself up on a program and monitor yourself because no one is doing it for you. I'm going to give you a few tools that dietitians and other weight counselors sometimes use to set up the right plan for each client. You don't have to use all the tools or answer every question. If you like, choose just one or two exercises that will help you learn enough about yourself and your personal habits to develop a sensible weight-management plan you can follow.

From now on, you're both counselor *and* client. Like any good weight-management counselor, the more you know about your own behavior, your own likes and dislikes, and your own weight background, the easier it will be to help yourself make smart lifestyle changes. Here are some of the first questions a counselor might ask:

NutriTip
The first step in creating a weight-management plan is to learn everything you can about yourself and about your eating and exercise habits because the next step is changing some of them. Once you're aware of any problems that are getting in your way, you can start taking steps to solve them.

➤ Do you have a family history of being overweight? You want to be sure you're setting realistic weight goals given your genetic background.

➤ When did your overeating begin? Did a particular physical or emotional event trigger the overeating that contributed to your weight gain?

➤ Has your weight fluctuated over time? When and how much? Be sure you're not just jumping back on the weight-loss roller coaster. This time you want to commit to a lifelong plan of healthier living.

➤ What kind of diets have you experienced in the past? List them on a piece of paper, along with what you liked and didn't like about each one. Circle your "likes" so that the features you enjoyed and think might fit into your new plan will stand out. You might find some patterns worth repeating.

➤ What do you think works for you? What aspects of losing weight have you most enjoyed in the past? The structure of a preplanned diet? Eating a certain type of food? The anticipation of buying new clothes? Getting back into a sport you once enjoyed?

71

➤ What doesn't work for you? What aspects of dieting have you hated in the past? Trying to squeeze in gym time on working days? Eating a certain type of food? There's no point repeating any patterns or using any strategies that absolutely failed you in the past.

Habits Are Habit Forming

The more information you have about yourself and your eating habits, the better able you'll be to come up with a realistic food plan. Do you

➤ Eat at random times?

➤ Skip meals?

➤ Eat on the run?

➤ Wait more than five hours before eating?

➤ Eat quickly?

➤ Snack constantly?

➤ Eat when you're not hungry? Why?

➤ Eat late at night?

➤ Go food shopping when you're hungry?

No Weigh!
Don't be too hard on yourself if change doesn't happen as quickly as you want it. Overeating is a tough habit to kick, and it takes time and a lot of effort to get used to new routines.

NutriTip
When you're not paying attention to what you're eating, you can go through the day mindlessly shoveling food in your mouth and never really know how much you ate. It's also easy to forget about food you eat on the run. The way to break these habits and stop overeating is to slow down and start planning and scheduling your meals and snacks.

If you answered yes to any of these questions, I won't report you to the diet police. I will tell you that any time you're not really paying attention to what you eat or you wait until you're starving to eat, you're in danger of overeating. With practice and patience and a plan, you can break bad habits and put new ones in their place.

How Did You Get Here?

Some people can shed enormous amounts of weight just by making a few lifestyle changes. You might be totally unaware of the eating behavior that's keeping you weighty. You have to know what needs to be changed before you can change it. Check off any situations in the My Weight-Loss Challenges Checklist you think might be contributing to your state of overweight.

My Weight-Loss Challenges Checklist

Check off all items that you think might contribute to your eating problems.

- ❏ Eating too much food
- ❏ Eating the wrong kinds of foods at home
- ❏ Eating out
- ❏ Eating fast foods
- ❏ Pressure to overeat from family
- ❏ Not enough time to prepare healthful foods
- ❏ Snacking frequently or constantly
- ❏ Emotional eating from anger, anxiety, or depression
- ❏ Eating from boredom
- ❏ Eating from loneliness
- ❏ Quitting smoking
- ❏ Other lifestyle change
- ❏ Reduced activity

What Are You Eating?

Dietitians call the next easy quiz a Food Frequency Questionnaire. After you fill it out, you'll have a better idea of how balanced or imbalanced your diet is. Do you eat a lot of meat? sugar? salt? Is your diet especially high in fat? If you haven't been paying attention to your diet up to this point, you might be surprised at what you find. Write down the number of times each week you eat each food or write N for never or R for rarely, if ever.

If you often eat foods in Group 1 of the Food Frequency Questionnaire, your diet might be too high in fat. Foods in Group 2 are loaded with sugar and possibly with fat, too. If you eat a lot of foods in Group 3, your diet might be too high in salt from sodium. Even though salt has no calories, a diet high in salt could mean you eat too many processed convenience foods and might not be getting enough vitamins, minerals, and fiber in your diet.

NutriTip
Foods that are high in sugar and fat are often called "empty calorie" foods because they provide a lot of calories but not much in the way of important nutrients such as vitamins and minerals.

No Weigh!
Stop picking on yourself! If you're criticizing yourself for not losing weight fast enough or not working out hard enough, ask yourself if you would say the same thing, the same way, to a friend. If not, you're probably not giving yourself constructive criticism.

Food Frequency Questionnaire

Write down the number of times each week you eat each food or write N for never or R for rarely, if ever.

Group 1

Beef	_____
Butter or margarine	_____
Olive oil or other vegetable oil	_____
Pork	_____
Whole milk	_____
Cheese	_____
Cream	_____
Pastries, cookies, or cakes	_____
Gravies/sauces	_____
Regular ice cream	_____

Group 2

Cakes	_____
Pastries	_____
Cookies	_____
Non-diet soft drinks	_____
Candy	_____
Sweetened cereals	_____

Group 3

Prepared frozen meals	_____
Canned soups	_____
Canned vegetables	_____
Frankfurters, cold cuts, ham, sausages	_____
Snack foods such as chips, crackers, nuts, and pretzels	_____
Pickles, relishes, and olives	_____
Smoked or canned fish	_____

What's Your Plan?

Almost without exception, a successful weight-loss plan has to include a change in your eating habits and a change in your activity level—not to mention a change in the attitude and behavior that keeps you overweight. If you joined a group weight-loss program, a plan would be laid out for you. Even the most flexible plan would provide a framework within which you would work. You're going to provide that structure yourself.

What's most important is that you like your plan. You have to wake up and live with your new plan every day and that's why it's worth putting some time and thought into it before you start. It's just like people. If you don't like your plan, you'll just find excuses to avoid it.

The first thing to do is target the behavior you most need to change. Is it your eating habits or your lack of activity that's holding you back? Is it your attitude or your crazy schedule that gets in the way? You might want to attack from all sides, and that's fine if you move slowly. Don't be tempted to change too much, too soon. Whatever you do, don't overwhelm yourself to the point that you get frustrated and have to give up.

Advice from Losers

"I come from a heavy family that had typical 1950s eating habits—bad! I'm barely 5'7" and by the time I was 38, I weighed 215 pounds. I work in food service so I became aware when the trend was toward healthier foods. But I had no idea what it meant to eat a balanced diet. I bought a book and figured out what I needed to do from tables and guidelines. I never went on a diet. I just ate right and exercised. I started walking, then started jogging. I lost 70 pounds over 10 months and dropped 8 pant sizes. I had to buy all new clothes and I enjoyed that. That was the payoff. That and the fact that I'm 45 and in the best shape I've been in since high school."

—Tom T.

You can start your fitness program right here, right now, before you even have any kind of real plan. You can do that by taking a look at the habits and eating patterns you outlined previously and picking one area where you can either introduce a single new, healthy habit into your life or start breaking an old self-destructive habit. For instance, you can decide to sit down and eat lunch at a regular, scheduled time at least three days a week, beginning right now. You can decide to go for an early evening walk every night after dinner instead of immediately plopping down in front of the TV as soon as the dishes are done.

You're Not Alone

You have to be your own cheerleader. You have to get out of bed each morning and psych yourself up to meet the daily challenge of losing weight and keeping it off. (I know. I know. Some days it's enough to just meet the challenge of getting up and out of bed!) Morning is a good time to prepare yourself for any stressful situations that might come up during that day and trigger you to overeat. Take some time to come up with some real solutions in advance of any problems you're able to anticipate. Planning helps. Really!

We all need to find some support outside ourselves. Don't be afraid to ask all the significant others and maybe some not-so-significant others in your life for help. Family members, friends, work associates, and anyone and everyone you live with should be aware of what you're trying to do and how they can help you. Be specific when you explain what you're trying to do and what you want them to do.

Who are the friends and family members you normally turn to for support? It's better to turn to the parent or brother or sister or friend who has been supportive in the past. Whatever you do, don't set yourself up for disappointment by trying to get support from someone who can't give it.

It might seem a little odd at first to write down the names of your family and friends (use the Supporters Worksheet if you want). After all, you *know* who they are! Losing weight can sometimes be a lonely and frustrating experience, and that's when it can be helpful to have a reminder at hand of the people you can count on for help. Just looking over a list of names of people who love and support you can help you get over the feeling of isolation.

Supporters Worksheet

Supporter	How He or She Can Help

Beyond your immediate circle of family and friends is a world full of people who can provide support and help fight the isolation of trying to lose weight on your own. If you know at least one other person who wants to lose weight, you can form an informal alliance to help each other. I once counseled two young women who did *everything* together to lose weight. They first met at work and started eating lunch together, and they grew into an effective weight-loss support team. They started eating out together and cooking low-fat meals at one or the other's home. When one's gym membership expired, she joined the other one's gym. They even acquired nutritional counseling together.

You might even consider forming your own small weight-loss group of maybe six or eight members and holding informal meetings in your home. You can solicit members at your gym, at your workplace, or by posting signs at a supermarket or community center. You don't need a specific agenda; gather together enough people who are obsessed with food and dieting, and there will always be something to talk about! To make it work and keep it going, you should have a definite time and place to meet each week.

> **No Weigh!**
> Don't let a friend's progress, or lack of it, hold you back or discourage you from your own fitness goals. Everyone is different and everyone loses weight and gets in shape at a different pace.

Any Problems?

A good weight-loss counselor evaluates your program from time to time to see if you need an adjustment. You can self-monitor by taking a little time each week to ask yourself these questions:

➤ Are you satisfied with your program as it is?

➤ Are you sticking to your plan?

➤ How's your emotional state (positive or negative)?

➤ Are you running into any obstacles such as lack of time?

➤ Is your support system holding up?

➤ Are you experimenting with new foods?

The Least You Need to Know

➤ Losing weight on your own takes a lot of self-motivation and readiness to change.

➤ It's a good idea to assess your family weight history, your eating and exercise habits, and your willingness to make lifestyle changes before you draw up a weight-loss plan. Use the worksheets and questionnaires in this chapter to perform an honest assessment.

➤ Be sure to monitor yourself as you go along and make any changes necessary to keep yourself on track.

➤ Surround yourself with supportive people and ask for help if you need it.

Part 3
Small Steps You Can Take Right Now

This is the part of the book where you finally start working on yourself and take the necessary steps to start developing a plan for managing your weight. You'll find out if this is really a good time for you to think about losing weight, figure out how much weight you can reasonably expect to lose, and start setting goals.

You'll start keeping a food diary to keep track of what and when and why you eat. Then you'll analyze your diary to figure out where you can make improvements in your food choices and eating patterns. You'll find easy-to-follow menus in this part, and you'll find easy ways to adjust them to suit your own personal taste and eating style. You're on your way!

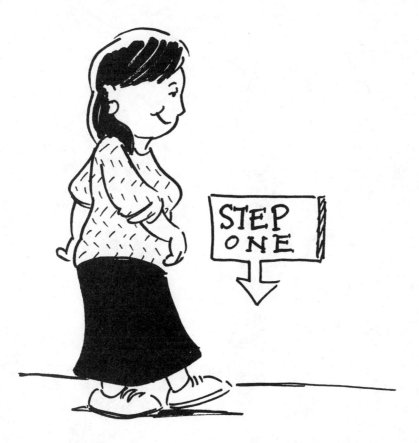

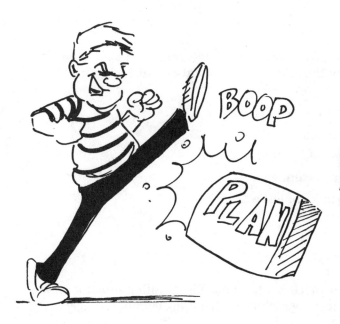

Chapter 8

Kick-Start Your Personal Plan

In This Chapter

➤ Getting off to a good start

➤ Changing your ways

➤ Setting short-term and long-term goals

➤ Small steps you can take right now

You've stuck your toe in the water and now you're ready to dive in. Good for you! This chapter gives you tools and tips for setting reasonable weight loss goals and living a healthier life.

Getting Off on the Right Foot

Losing weight isn't an all-or-nothing proposition. You can't just stop eating, and you can't expect to change your eating and exercise habits overnight. That's too drastic. It won't last. That's why fad diets don't work. It's too much change too soon, without any thought about whether a plan is right for you. What you can do is surround yourself with the tools you need to start making permanent changes in your life and keep using those tools. The best place to start is with yourself. Then you can move on to food and exercise.

Check Your Attitude

Attitude isn't everything when it comes to losing weight, but it counts for a lot. How do you feel about losing weight? If most of the following statements are true for you, you have the right attitude:

➤ I'm looking forward to shedding those extra pounds.

➤ I don't feel angry because I have to lose weight.

➤ I think losing weight will make me feel better.

➤ I think losing weight will make me healthier.

➤ I don't expect anyone to like me more or less when I lose weight.

➤ I'm losing weight for me.

Be Prepared

One of the best things you can do for yourself is know your trigger eating situations and be prepared to avoid them. Here are a few suggestions for handling common triggers:

➤ Don't carry change in your pocket for vending machines. If you're in the habit of wandering over to the snack machine when you get a break at work or school, be prepared by being unprepared.

➤ Brush your teeth between meals. This old trick is one of my favorites for breaking an "oversnacking" habit. Your dentist will love it, too!

➤ Eat some small amount of food before you go to a party or a restaurant. It's okay to save up your calories during the day on special occasions when you know you're going out, but don't go anywhere starving.

➤ Bring your own food. Do what my mother does. She takes little plastic bags filled with sliced apples, cut-up vegetables, and sunflower seeds to the movies so she won't be tempted to buy candy or other junk food. She also takes these little bags with her on car trips and bus trips and whenever she knows she'll be away from healthy food for any length of time.

> **NutriTip**
> Carry your own healthy foods with you to work, to school, on long rides, to the movies, and any other time you might be tempted to eat from a vending machine. Even if you still indulge in a candy bar or other junk food, at least you'll have something healthier to go with it.

Time for a Change

Change doesn't happen quickly because most habits are so ingrained in our day-to-day lives that our actions become automatic. Real change only happens in stages over time. Dr. James Prochaska, a psychologist at the University of Rhode Island, actually defined six stages of change we all go through before a problem no longer exists. At least five of these stages apply to anyone who's ever tried to lose weight.

When you know which stage of change you're in, it's easier to know what you should do next to prepare yourself to lose weight. You could be at any one of these stages right now—and you might not move gracefully from one stage to the next. You might go back and forth between two stages until you're ready to move forward again. Here are Prochaska's stages of change and what they mean when you're trying to lose weight:

> **Guru's Corner**
> "Most people blow it a few times before they succeed at any type of change. But you can't let fear of failure stop you from trying again. If you try to lose weight and give up within a month, you're still twice as likely to succeed over the next six months than someone who didn't try at all."
>
> —James O. Prochaska, Ph.D., professor of psychology at the University of Rhode Island and author of *Changing for Good* (Avon Books, 1994)

1. **Precontemplation.** You're not even thinking about losing weight. You think it's hopeless or unnecessary. Maybe you don't think your weight is hazardous to your health. Or you're in that blissful state of denial where you think you can still lose weight as easily as you could when you were young. Or you don't believe it's possible to lose weight. Someone gave you this book, but you haven't really begun to think seriously about losing weight. You're not ready to start planning any lifestyle changes yet.

2. **Contemplation.** You've just started to think, "Maybe I need to lose weight," or even, "I better stop gaining weight right now." You start thinking about how much effort it will take and whether it's worth the effort. The problem with this stage is that you can stay stuck in it for a long time. Years, even.

3. **Preparation.** You've decided to do something about your weight. You're in the planning stage, looking into different methods. You got the name of your friend's nutritionist, or you took a tour of your local gym. You took a small but important step.

4. **Action.** At this stage of the weight-loss game, you're finally, actually doing something. You joined the gym, you bought the book, you made an appointment with a weight loss counselor. You've loaded the fridge with low-fat foods. You took the big step. You're actually changing things. This stage is when you should go slowly so you don't overwhelm yourself with too much change at once.

5. **Maintenance.** You've made your lifestyle changes and you're sticking with them. Handled properly, this stage can last for the rest of your life. Here's where you have to be careful not to get too overconfident or give in to old, destructive habits such as negative self-talk and self-blame when you have occasional lapses.

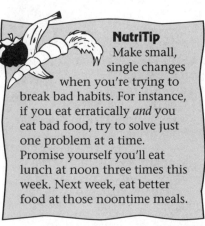

NutriTip
Make small, single changes when you're trying to break bad habits. For instance, if you eat erratically *and* you eat bad food, try to solve just one problem at a time. Promise yourself you'll eat lunch at noon three times this week. Next week, eat better food at those noontime meals.

6. **Termination.** No, it doesn't mean that you lie down and die now. It means you're out of the cycle of change. Nothing more needs to be done; you've changed. However, I'm not sure that weight loss ever gets beyond maintenance for some of us. I think we get to Stage 5 and stay there. If we stick it out, maintenance gets easier with time. If you get to a point where you feel sure that you'll no longer be tempted to return to old, self-defeating habits, you can safely say you've reached the stage of termination.

What Are Your Goals?

Setting goals, writing them down, and monitoring them as you go along are all essential steps that will help you get fit. The three types of goals are

➤ Long-term

➤ Intermediate-term

➤ Short-term

Long-term goals represent the end results or the bigger picture, as they say. One of your long-term goals is the total amount of weight you want to lose to get to a healthier weight.

NutriTip
Keep your focus on the small, daily goals that will help you change your eating and exercise habits and bring you closer to your larger, long-term goals.

Intermediate goals are somewhat long-term but more realistic to think about for the time being. A realistic intermediate weight-loss goal is a percentage, say 10 percent, of your long-term weight-loss goal. If your long-term goal is to lose 60 pounds, your intermediate goal could be to lose 6 pounds.

Short-term goals are the ones you can realize in a short period of time, such as losing a pound in a week. You can realistically focus on these goals every day. As time goes on, you'll find yourself updating your short-term goals and setting new ones. Your short-term goals are all the steps that get you to your long-term goal.

Sometimes it's also a good idea to set very-short-term goals. These goals are shorter than short-term. Often they satisfy a need to do something *right now*. For instance, a very-short-term food goal is to add more vegetables to your meal for dinner tonight. A very-short-term activity goal might be to walk to the market to buy the vegetables instead of taking the car. No long-term commitments, just one-day goals.

Not Just a Number

Your goals for losing weight and getting fit are much more than just the number of pounds you want to lose or the number of pounds you want to weigh. Fill out the Short-Term Goal Organizer in this chapter. In it, you'll be setting

➤ **Exercise goals.** You set these goals to increase your activity one way or another. If you're not exercising at all, your short-term goal might be to walk around the block every morning before you go to work. Your intermediate goal could be to switch from walking to jogging within a month. Your long-term goal might then be to jog three miles a day at least three days a week.

➤ **Food goals.** These goals include your plans to change what you eat and how much you eat and could even include the practice of learning more about good nutrition. Your long-term goal probably includes eating less food. Your intermediate goal might be to practice portion control. Your short-term goal could be to eat only single helpings of even your most favorite foods, starting right now.

➤ **Psychological goals.** These are your goals for changing the way you think about yourself, about food, about exercise, and about being a healthy person. Perhaps your long-term goal is to improve your self-esteem. Your intermediate goal might be to break the habit of negative self-talk. Your short-term goal might be to buy a book on the subject or seek psychological counseling to help you make changes you can't make on your own.

➤ **Behavioral goals.** If one of your long-term goals is to improve your overall eating habits, one of your intermediate goals could be to eat more slowly. Setting and reaching short-term goals such as chewing your food completely before you swallow it, or putting your fork down between mouthfuls, will help you get to your intermediate goal of slowing down.

Whether your current goals are focused on food, exercise, behavior, or mind-set, they should all have certain traits in common. When you set your goals, long or short, be sure they're realistic. If you say you want to go to the gym to work out three times a week, make sure you have time in your schedule. Make your goals as specific as possible. Instead of just saying, "I want to be thinner," say "I want to lose 15 pounds" or "I want to knock two inches off my waistline." When your goals are specific, it's easier to come up with a real plan to meet them. When you have a specific goal, you can measure your progress and see exactly how close you are to that goal. It's also a good idea to give each goal a realistic time frame or a deadline. Again, this helps you measure how close you are to your goal and whether it's realistic.

> **No Weigh!**
> Don't promise yourself you'll go to the gym five times a week if you don't really have time in your schedule. Don't say "I'll never eat another potato chip" unless you've suddenly lost your taste for them. Instead, say "I'll get to the gym at least twice this week" and "I'll try not to eat potato chips today."

Short-Term Goal Organizer

(Note that the blank lines are for additional goals.)

Area	Goal	Time Frame	How to Get There	How to Measure
Food	_____	_____	_____	_____
Food	_____	_____	_____	_____
Food	_____	_____	_____	_____
Exercise	_____	_____	_____	_____
Exercise	_____	_____	_____	_____
Exercise	_____	_____	_____	_____
State-of-mind	_____	_____	_____	_____
State-of-mind	_____	_____	_____	_____
State-of-mind	_____	_____	_____	_____
Behavior	_____	_____	_____	_____
Behavior	_____	_____	_____	_____
Behavior	_____	_____	_____	_____

_____

_____

_____

What Can You Lose?

The healthy weight ranges in Table 8.1 show another version of the healthy weight chart from Chapter 2, "Why You're Weighty." Remember, the entire range is not your healthy weight range. Your healthy weight falls somewhere in this range depending on your exact height, how much of your weight is fat, and the location of fat on your body. The lower end of the range generally applies to women and the higher end to men. Use this chart to set your own healthy weight goal and when you do, consider the following:

➤ The amount of weight you need to lose

➤ Your level of physical activity

➤ Any medical problems or concerns

➤ Your emotional state

➤ Your dieting history

Table 8.1 Healthy Weight Ranges

Height*	Weight (in Pounds)**
4'10"	91–119
4'11"	94–124
5'0"	97–128
5'1"	101–132
5'2"	104–137
5'3"	107–141
5'4"	111–146
5'5"	114–150
5'6"	118–155
5'7"	121–160
5'8"	125–164
5'9"	129–169
5'10"	132–174
5'11"	136–179
6'0"	140–184
6'1"	144–189
6'2"	148–195
6'3"	152–200
6'4"	156–205
6'5"	160–211
6'6"	164–216

*Without shoes

**Without clothes

Source: Dietary Guidelines for Americans, 1995 ed., U.S. Department of Agriculture, U.S. Department of Health and Human Services.

Now, use the Healthy Weight Goal worksheet on the following page to write down your healthy weight goal here so you can refer to it later and set your long-term weight-loss goals and intermediate goals.

Healthy Weight Goal Worksheet

Healthy Weight Goal: _____

Subtract your healthy weight from today's weight. That's your long-term, healthy weight-loss goal. Write it down here:

Today's Date: _____

Today's Weight: _____

Healthy Weight: _____

Long-Term Healthy Weight Loss Goal: _____

Remember that it's important to have long-term, intermediate-term, and short-term weight-loss goals. No matter what your long-term weight loss goal is, your intermediate goal should be to lose no more than five to ten percent of your current weight in a reasonable amount of time. For example, someone who weighs 150 pounds right now with a long-term healthy weight goal of 120 pounds will have an intermediate goal to lose between 7 and 15 pounds. Calculate your intermediate goal and estimated goal date and write it down here:

Intermediate Healthy Weight Loss Goal: _____

Losing one pound a week, I can reach that goal by this date: _____

If you lose a little more than a pound a week, you'll reach your intermediate weight goal that much sooner. However, rather than set yourself up for disappointment, set a goal date based on just a pound a week.

Your short-term, healthy weight-loss goal is always to lose about one pound a week until you reach your intermediate, healthy weight goal. Write down your short-term goal weights and goal dates for the next few weeks:

Goal Weight: _____

By _____

Goal Weight: _____

By _____

Goal Weight: _____

By _____

Goal Weight: _____

By _____

A Step at a Time

You're on your way! If you've gotten this far, answered all those questions, and filled in all those blanks, you're prepared to start getting fit. From this point on, you're going to be taking real steps toward reaching your weight goals. In the next chapter, you'll learn how to keep a food diary, one of the most important first steps in developing a healthier food and lifestyle plan. As you move along through this book, you'll be fine-tuning your plan as you learn more about eating well, exercising your excess weight off, and exorcising any demons that get in your way.

Meanwhile, you might already know a lot about healthy eating, exercising, and improving your mindset, even if you don't always put it all into practice. If so, the following section is a refresher course for you. If you don't have even a clue how to put together a healthy meal or motivate yourself to work out, you can start living a healthier lifestyle right now just by picking up a few of these basic tips.

> **No Weigh!**
> You can't always lose weight according to schedule. Remember that goals are not absolute and are always subject to adjustment and change.

> **NutriTip**
> Make every day an eating adventure. Try an exotic new fruit or vegetable. Learn how to use fresh herbs in your cooking. Try out a new kitchen gadget. Be a vegetarian for a day. Pick out a new cookbook that will add a little spice to your food life.

Let's Eat!

You'll soon be designing your own personal food plan, but meanwhile, here are a few general tips to lead you down the road toward healthier eating habits:

➤ Try something different—anything! Experiment with new foods to get accustomed to the idea of change.

➤ Start planning your meals and snacks so you can begin to break the habit of random eating.

➤ Ask the butcher at the supermarket to help you choose leaner cuts of meat.

➤ Eat more fresh fruits and vegetables. If you're not used to preparing fresh produce, look for a cookbook that shows you how. (Check Appendix B, "Your Best Resources," for a list of recommended cookbooks.)

➤ Eat a variety of foods at every meal and even at snack times. For instance, rather than a fistful of crackers, have a couple of crackers with a small piece of cheese and an apple.

➤ When you're tempted to eat for any reason other than hunger, stop first and look up the number of calories and grams of fat in the food you have in mind. Ask yourself whether it's worth it. This is one of the best uses I can imagine for calorie and fat gram charts and one reason you'll find such a chart in the back of this book. If you end up eating for reasons other than hunger, at least you'll have learned something about the food you're putting in your mouth.

➤ If you have a hard time eating "just one" of anything, buy small, individual, or single-serving packages. You won't save money, but you'll probably save calories.

➤ When you go out to a restaurant, stay away from "all you can eat" buffets.

Move It!

There are a lot of ways to burn extra calories in your day-to-day life and some small steps you can take while you're still thinking about a more serious exercise program. Here are just a few:

➤ When you drive to work or to the movies or to the mall, leave your car at the far end of the parking lot so you're forced to do a little walking back and forth.

➤ If you find yourself wanting to eat when you're not hungry, take a walk. Go out in the garden. If you can't go out, move around the house with a vacuum cleaner or a dust mop in your hands instead of a cookie. Wash your windows or wipe down your cabinets. Although these aren't serious calorie-burning exercises, they can help move you past a food craving.

No Weigh!
Unfortunately, sex doesn't burn as many calories as you might think, even if you work up a sweat. In fact, an orgasm burns only about a calorie and a half. Of course, if you're aggressive about sex and go at it for at least an hour every day, you might work off an extra pound or two a month. But no promises!

➤ If you're not already a member, take a free tour of your local gym or stop by your YMCA or YWCA for a catalog of exercise classes. While you're at it, check out a local dance school.

➤ When you have a choice, take the stairs instead of the escalator or elevator. At the end of the day, extra activities such as this add up and can contribute to weight loss.

➤ Get a checkup. If you're over 35 and haven't been exercising, make an appointment with your doctor for a complete physical. Discuss your weight loss plans and let the doctor know your exercise intentions.

Get Psyched!

To lose weight, you'll need a lot of motivation and "continuing education." Here are a few ways to get both:

➤ If you overeat for emotional reasons (and who doesn't?), start thinking about new ways to relax. Check out a local yoga school or day spa and see what they have to offer in the way of relaxation techniques.

➤ Browse through the self-help section of your bookstore and look for books that deal with familiar issues.

➤ Start gathering your support team. Let everyone know what you're about to do.

➤ Think about how you're going to feel when you're fit.

➤ Pick up a new health or fitness magazine.

➤ Subscribe to a health and nutrition newsletter. Here are a few good ones:

Consumer Reports on Health
(800) 234-2188

Mayo Clinic Health Letter
(800) 333-9037

Tufts University Diet & Nutrition Letter
(800) 274-7581

The Least You Need to Know

➤ A positive attitude is essential when you're planning to make lifestyle changes.

➤ Change is a slow process that occurs in steps. Permanent change never happens quickly.

➤ When it comes to setting weight-loss goals, think long-term but act short-term.

➤ Take small steps, one at a time, to change your eating and exercise habits. Don't overwhelm yourself by trying to do too much at once.

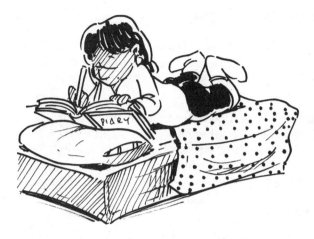

Chapter 9

Dear Diary...

In This Chapter
➤ Why it's important to keep a food diary
➤ Deciding what to put in your diary
➤ What you can learn from your diary
➤ Using your diary as a tool for change

It probably won't surprise you to hear that, when asked, most people say they eat less food than they actually eat. It's not that we lie (although the state of denial can be a great place to live)! It's just hard to keep track of every cookie you grab as you run out the door or even to remember what you had for breakfast this morning. It's easy to get confused about how much you actually eat, especially if you're not always dishing out your own food.

Keeping a food diary is the best way to watch what you eat. At the end of the day, you have right in front of you all the information you need about how, what, and why you eat. From there, you can begin to make improvements.

This chapter explains what a food diary is, how to keep one, and how to analyze your diet. You'll learn how to use the information in your diary to change the way you eat and, if necessary, how to change the way you think.

What Exactly Is a Food Diary?

Starting your food diary is probably the most important first step you can take toward designing a food plan that will work for you. It's not only a written record of how you eat right now, but a tool you can use later to measure your progress and maintain your weight loss.

NutriTip
Keeping a food diary could motivate you to eat less from day one. When you know you have to write down everything you put in your mouth, you might think twice about overeating and eating junk food.

Guru's Corner
"You already know that whatever you've been doing to lose weight hasn't been working. But you may not know why. Your food diary can point out things you never knew about how and why you eat. Once you become aware of your weak areas, you can start making useful changes and setting real goals."

—Mindy Hermann, M.P.H., R.D., President, The Hermann Group, and former spokesperson for the American Dietetic Association

At first, you'll use your food diary to learn about your current eating habits. You'll see how much and how often you eat. Scary as it sounds, writing down what you eat might turn out to be your best motivator for losing weight. At the end of the day, when everything you ate is right there in your face, you'll be highly inspired to do something about it!

You can use your food diary to record more than what you eat. It can be a record of your different emotions and the day-to-day situations that trigger problem eating. Those triggers are different for everyone, and your diary will make you more aware of the ones that affect you. You can also use your food diary to record exercise and any other activities that are part of your effort to have a healthier lifestyle. You can write notes to yourself in the margin or copy inspirational messages.

Take a week or so to learn about your eating habits before you try to change them. What kind of foods do you eat? How much of those foods do you eat? How often do you eat them? Why are you eating? Your diary will give you clear answers to these questions. Once you have the answers, it's easy to design an eating plan that suits your particular tastes and lifestyle. Keep a food diary, and you're also more likely to make the types of lifestyle changes you need to lose weight and keep it off.

While you're keeping your food diary, read Chapters 10 through 14. In these chapters, you'll find basic information about good nutrition to help you analyze your diary at the end of the week. Once you have a better understanding of what it means to eat balanced, healthful meals, you'll have an easier time making adjustments to your own diet.

How to Keep a Food Diary

Pick some sort of notebook to use as your diary. It can be a beautiful blank book, a daily calendar, or a few pieces of note paper stapled together. (For now, you can use the food diary provided at the end of this section.) Lined paper is more orderly, but anything that's easy to carry and has enough space for at least a week's worth of entries will do. You'll probably need a wide piece of paper or a double page to accommodate all your categories.

Across the top of each page of your diary, write the following categories:

➤ Time

➤ Food

➤ Amount

➤ Reason

➤ Location

➤ Partner

➤ Time Spent Eating

If you also want to use your food diary as an exercise log, add another column at the top of the page and simply label it "Exercise." That is good enough if all you need to log right now is something such as "20-min. run" or "Walked around block." If you're starting a major exercise program and want to keep track of a number of different workouts, you need to use the back side of each page or perhaps divide your book in half and log your exercise in a separate section.

Every time you eat, whether it's a full meal, a planned snack, or just a quick bite, record the following information:

➤ Under Time, write in the time of day you started eating.

➤ Under Food, enter the name of the food you ate. Enter only one food or drink on each line and break down the components of mixed foods. For instance, instead of writing "spaghetti and meatballs" on one line, write "spaghetti" on one line and "meatballs" on the next. If you made the spaghetti and meatballs yourself, you can also put the sauce on its own line because you know how much you used. If you're eating away from home, you probably have to record one amount of spaghetti and sauce on the same line. That's okay.

➤ Under Amount, fill in the weight or quantity of each food you listed in the food column. For

NutriTip
If you've never tried it before, it pays to spend a little time measuring your food before you eat to see just how much food you're really eating and to begin to understand standard serving sizes. Remember, this is just a temporary learning tool, not something you'll be doing for the rest of your life.

example, you might enter "12" for grapes, "3 ounces" for sliced ham, or "$^1/_2$ cup" for mashed potatoes. Be as accurate as possible without driving yourself nuts. Use food labels to help you figure out how much you eat. Whenever possible, at first, measure your food with standard kitchen measuring tools. Check food packaging for weights and measures.

➤ Under Reason, write your motivation for eating. Because your reason for eating might have something to do with the mood you're in, a wide range of answers is appropriate here. You might write in "hungry" or "bored" or "lonely" or any other reason why you chose to eat at that particular time.

➤ Under Location, fill in where you were when you were eating. It might be a restaurant, it might be at your dining room table, or it could be at a friend's house. It could also be leaning against the refrigerator, sitting in front of the TV, driving in your car, or walking around the mall, and these might be the habits you're looking to change.

➤ Under Partner, write down the names of anyone you were eating with. Different people can influence the type of foods you eat, and you need to be aware of that.

➤ Under Time Spent Eating, fill in the total amount of time, usually in minutes, you actually spent eating.

If you're fond of counting calories or fat grams, a food diary is certainly a good place to do it. Just leave an extra column on the side of each page for your numbers. Personally, I don't bother much with this kind of math unless I'm demonstrating the nutritional difference between, say, sour cream and fat-free sour cream. For those of you who enjoy the arithmetic of it all, Appendix A, "Calorie and Fat Chart for Selected Foods," contains calorie and fat grams for many common foods.

Your food diary will look something like the sample food diary:

Be consistent. Every day, write down what you eat, when you eat, the time you eat, and why you eat. It's best to record each meal and snack just before or after you eat it so you don't forget.

Be honest. Don't be afraid to write down each and every piece of food you eat. There's no reason to hide the information from yourself. Even if you don't record that candy bar, you'll know you ate it. If you let yourself forget, your scale will eventually remind you!

Be precise. Try to keep accurate records, but don't make yourself crazy. If you worry too much about exact times and measurements, you'll get frustrated and you might give up.

Be flexible. If you can't keep your diary for one day because your schedule interferes, start again the next day. If your diary is incomplete at the end of the day, fill in the blanks as best you can from memory.

As noted earlier, you can use any type of paper or notebook for your food diary. You can also make copies of the following blank diary page to carry individually or staple together like a booklet. Just do what's easiest for you.

Sample Food Diary

Time	Food	Amount	Reason	Location	Partner	Time Spent Eating
7:45	Bagel Cream cheese Coffee Peach	¹/₂ 2 tbsp. 2 cups 1	Breakfast	Kitchen	Joe	20 min.
10:30	Danish Coffee	1 1 cup	Bored	Desk at work	Self	2 min.
Noon	Pasta salad w/mixed vegetables Saltines Diet coke	2 cups 2 1 can	Lunch	Desk	Self	15 min.
3:30	Banana	1	Break	Desk	Self	1 min.
8:00	Red wine Swordfish Broccoli Olive oil Lettuce Tomato Ital. Bread Butter	2 glasses 1 steak 4 stalks 1 tbsp. 2 cups 4 wedges 3 slices 1 pat	Out to dinner	Dino's	Joe	1 hour

Gym: Treadmill, 20 minutes
Rower, 12 minutes.

Food Diary

Date:

Time	Food	Amount	Reason	Location	Partner	Time Spent Eating

Gym/Workout:

What Your Diary Tells You

Once you've kept records for at least five days (but preferably a week), it's time to analyze your diary to get a sense of how, why, and what you eat.

Take a good look at your eating habits and ask yourself a few basic questions:

➤ Am I actually hungry when I eat?

➤ Do I skip meals? (If you go longer than five hours without eating, you've skipped a meal.)

➤ Do I eat too often? (If something's going into your mouth every 45 minutes, that's probably too often.)

➤ Do I snack instead of sitting down to regular meals?

➤ Do I eat too fast? (If dinner's over in five minutes flat, the answer is "yes.")

➤ Do I undereat early in the day and then get ravenously hungry and overeat later?

➤ Do I eat in response to moods or mood swings?

NutriTip
In the beginning, keep a food diary for at least five days. These don't have to be five consecutive days, but they should be five days that represent the way you usually eat. At least one of these days should be a weekend day.

After you look at your overall patterns, look more closely at the specific types of food you eat. Do you

➤ Eat a balanced diet? If you eat a wide variety of foods from different food groups, including dairy, fruits, vegetables, cereals and other grains, and meat or meat substitutes, your diet is likely to be balanced.

➤ Eat the same foods all the time? Variety is key to a balanced diet, and trying new foods is one way to break old eating habits.

➤ Choose too many high-fat foods? Look for fried foods, fast foods, and frozen convenience foods as well as oils, butter, cheeses, and other naturally high-fat foods.

➤ Eat one large meal each day? Ideally, the amount of food you eat will be evenly divided into three meals and perhaps a snack or two throughout the day.

➤ Eat an overabundance of foods from any one food group? If, for instance, you eat a lot of carbohydrates in the form of bread, pasta, crackers, and other grain foods but fewer than five fruits and vegetables a day, your diet might be out of balance.

The reason I asked you to record "spaghetti" and "meatballs" separately when you were learning how to keep a diary is to highlight the different food groups. That way, when it comes time to analyze your diary, it's easier to see how balanced, or unbalanced, your diet really is. Do you eat too much meat? Too much bread? Not enough vegetables? The more "itemized" your diary, the easier it is to answer these questions.

No Weigh!
Stop keeping a food diary after three days if you don't like the process. Don't let it frustrate you to the point of giving up before you even get started!

It's possible that you overeat out of boredom or simply out of habit, and if that's the case, it might not be so difficult for you to make changes. It might just be a matter of breaking patterns in your daily routine such as walking in a different direction on your way to work so you don't pass a certain bakery. Maybe you have to find some new day-to-day activities that don't include eating. If your diary entries suggest you overeat for deeper emotional reasons, such as depression or anxiety, it's important that you deal with those issues before you worry too much about what and how you're eating. Review Chapter 4, "Heavy Thoughts," and then skip over to Part 6, "Mind Over Matter," for some help figuring out just what's bugging you and why you're turning to food for answers.

Breaking Bad Eating Habits

Once you've identified and evaluated your eating habits, it's time to figure out where you can make *small* changes and start shifting the patterns that aren't working for you. Remember: *You don't want to make any drastic changes or make too many changes at once.*

Here are some examples of typical eating patterns and suggestions for breaking the habit:

➤ Old pattern: You're a nibbler who eats a lot of mini-meals and snacks throughout the day.

New plan: Switch from random eating to three small meals at regular times and a couple of scheduled snacks each day.

➤ Old pattern: You eat three gigantic meals every day and that's it.

New plan: Eat a little less food at each meal.

➤ Old pattern: You frequently skip meals throughout the day and then eat too much at night.

New plan: Eat a small breakfast as early in the day as possible and a small lunch no more than five hours later. You can still eat a big dinner but might not be so ravenously hungry that you overeat.

➤ Old pattern: You eat too much junk food and often eat sweets and fatty snacks in place of real meals.

New plan: Plan three balanced meals a day, following each with a small serving of a favorite treat. Continue to have one or two small snacks between meals.

Advice from Losers

"I was horrified the first time I kept a food diary and analyzed it. I was eating a lot of food and eating all the time. No wonder I weighed more than 200 pounds! I've lost the weight but I know I could gain some of it back in no time flat. So the minute I feel out of control, I start another diary. And I take a small spiral notebook with me whenever I go on vacation or leave my normal life for more than a day. I actually enjoy it. I have every food diary I ever I wrote and I always refer to them. They're the true story of my life!"

—Meryl M.

You probably don't need me or your diary to point out the small, everyday routines that can sabotage your plan to lose weight. You know the ones I'm talking about: strolling to the vending machine every afternoon for a package of peanut-butter crackers or stopping every night on your way home from work to pick up a pint of ice cream.

The solutions? Change the route you take when you come home at night so you don't drive past the ice cream store. Walk in the opposite direction of the snack machine during your afternoon break. Don't just change cold turkey; prepare yourself. Keep a supply of frozen fruit bars in your freezer so you won't go back out for the ice cream. Take healthier snacks with you to work or school so you have a ready substitute for your usual junk food.

You can keep a food diary as long as you want, and you can put it down and pick it up again some other time. Start a new diary whenever you need a little help staying on track. Like any journal, a food diary is a memory-keeper. Save your diaries, and later, they'll be a reminder of where you were when you started and how far you've come.

The Least You Need to Know

> ➤ Keeping a food diary is an important first step in any weight loss plan.

> ➤ A food diary is a record of what you eat, when you eat, how much you eat, and why you eat.

> ➤ By keeping a food diary, you learn about your eating habits so you can concentrate on problem areas.

> ➤ Once you recognize the problem areas in your diet, you can take steps to change them.

> ➤ If keeping a food diary becomes a burden, put it away for a while.

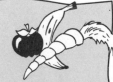

NutriTip
When you write in your food diary, include any positive feelings you have about yourself and your efforts at weight control. That way, your diary is more than just a record of how and why you eat. It also becomes a source of inspiration on low-confidence days and might help motivate you to get back on track.

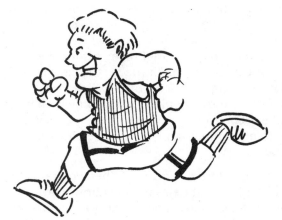

Chapter 10

Ready, Set, Go!

In This Chapter

➤ Figuring out your calorie count

➤ Easy-to-follow everyday menus

➤ Charting your success

➤ Calorie-free rewards and diversions

You know that when you want to lose weight, you can't just eat whatever and whenever you want. You have to maintain some kind of control. The real trick, however, is staying in control *and* enjoying yourself at the same time. Yes, it's possible!

If you're busy counting calories, keeping track of all your fat grams, and weighing yourself every day, you're probably not having much fun with food. This chapter shows you how to satisfy your need to monitor your numbers and at the same time take a somewhat freer approach to eating well.

How Much Can You Eat?

"How many calories can I have?" is a common question from dieters. Everyone knows this much: You want to burn more calories than you consume. If you eat fewer calories than you're eating now, you might lose weight. You already know that to lose one pound, you have to reduce calorie intake by 3,500 or burn off that many calories by exercising. Even though the number of calories consumed and burned is the basis of weight control, however, counting calories isn't a long-term solution for losing weight. That's because calorie counting is too restrictive for most people. You can only keep it up for so long. It's not always healthy, either. We become obsessed with numbers, begin thinking about food only as "fattening" or "nonfattening," and even stop eating certain healthy foods just because of their calorie counts.

No Weigh!
Don't be tempted to skip meals or eat only tiny amounts of food at meals when you're trying to lose weight. Eating too little food forces your body into "starvation mode." When your body thinks it's starving, it holds on to calories more tightly and this makes weight loss more difficult.

Don't get me wrong; calories *do* matter. When you're learning how to eat better, it helps to know how many calories are right for you. It also helps to know the number of calories in the foods you eat so you can compare and make choices among different brands and styles of similar foods. If you get the same amount of protein and calcium in a 100-calorie yogurt as in a 250-calorie yogurt, and you enjoy the flavor of both yogurts, why eat extra calories? But watching calories is only one part of getting fit. To use the preceding example, if you don't want to eat low-cal yogurt because you don't like artificial sweetener, you should be free to eat the regular variety and not worry that you'll gain weight as a result.

Calculating Calories

For those of you who like diet math, I'm including formulas such as the one that follows for figuring out how many calories you can eat every day to maintain a healthy weight. Remember, however, that formulas are limited. The results are simply guidelines, not absolute numbers to live by. For each and every one of us, there is a range of calories within which we can successfully lose and maintain weight.

NutriTip
A healthy food plan, even one that's designed to help you lose weight, should always include at least 1,200 calories. Below that, your metabolism might slow down and you won't get enough of the nutrients you need to stay healthy.

How much you can eat and maintain your healthy weight depends on how much energy your body uses. There's a minimum number of calories you *must* eat to have enough energy to be healthy. It's easy to figure out that one. Just take your healthy weight (if you don't know it, choose a mid-range weight from Table 8.1, Healthy Weight Ranges, in Chapter 8) and multiply it by 10 if you're a female and 11 if you're male.

_____ × _____ = _____

(Healthy weight) × (10 or 11) = Your basic calorie needs

That's just the number of calories your body needs to do its basic work. It's called the basal metabolic rate or resting metabolic rate. This is the amount of energy required just to keep your heart pumping, your brain thinking, your liver detoxifying, and all your other body systems working at full speed.

Now you have to figure out how many calories you need for digesting and absorbing nutrients from food. (Yes! You burn calories when you digest and absorb the food you eat.) Add your basic calorie needs and your activity calorie needs and multiply the total by 10 percent (0.10).

_____ + _____ × 0.10 = _____

Basic cal. needs + Activity cal. needs × 0.10 = Calories for digestion

Now figure out how many calories you need for any activity you do above and beyond sleeping. Figure out your activity level from the following descriptions and then multiply your basic calorie needs by the percentage that matches your activity level.

➤ Sedentary (20 percent): You sit, drive, lie down, or stand in one place for most of the day and don't do any type of exercise. Multiply by 0.20.

➤ Lightly active (30 percent): You walk but not for more than two hours a day. Multiply by 0.30.

➤ Moderately active (40 percent): You do very little sitting. Instead, you garden, dance, do a lot of housework, or take exercise classes. Multiply by 0.40.

➤ Very active (50 percent): You're active in a physical sport or a labor-intensive job such as construction work. Multiply by 0.50.

_____ × _____ = _____

Basic calorie needs × Percent activity level = Activity calorie needs

The last step is to add your basic calorie needs, your activity calorie needs, and your calorie needs for digestion and absorption of nutrients from food. Voilà! This figure represents your total energy needs in calories.

Basic calorie needs _____ +

Calories for digestion _____ +

Active calorie needs _____

Total daily calorie need = _____

NutriTip
The heavier you are, the more calories you burn. That's because your extra weight forces you to work harder at everything you do. That's why the closer you get to those last ten pounds, the harder it is to shake off the weight.

This final figure is the number of calories you can eat every day to maintain a healthy weight. If you're trying to get to your healthy weight (that is, you're trying to lose weight), you can use this figure as a guide to the *maximum* number of calories you eat on any given day. The actual number of calories that works for you depends on how much exercise you decide to do when you start making lifestyle changes.

More Than Calories

Even though everyone makes such a big deal out of it, counting calories is really only a small part of losing and maintaining weight. Think about it. There are plenty of overweight people who can recite the number of calories in every known food product—but they can't shake off the weight!

Because everyone's different, not everyone loses or maintains weight at the same calorie level. Even two people who are the same height and same general frame size and who get equal amounts of exercise have different calorie requirements because their bodies handle the calories differently.

No Weigh!
Never set a daily calorie level that provides less than ten calories per pound of your current weight. For instance, if you weigh 150 pounds, your average calorie count for the day should be no less than 1,500.

When you set a calorie limit for yourself, do yourself a favor and set a range. Trying to hit a precise calorie count each day would drive you crazy in terms of food choices, quantities, and menu planning. If you decide you can lose or maintain weight on 1,600 calories a day, make that 1,500 to 1,700 calories. That gives you some leeway on days when you want to eat something special or you feel hungrier than usual.

Simple Menus for Success

My favorite approach to healthy eating is to develop menu plans that represent both a balanced diet and a reasonable number of calories. If you and I were in a private counseling session, I would go over your food diary, ask you about the types of food you like to eat, and find out about your eating patterns. Armed with that information, I'd develop a series of calorie-adjusted menu plans for you to follow—but now you can do that for yourself.

Learn by Example

By following my daily menus and then using their example to develop similar menus of your own, you'll soon know exactly what it means to eat 1,400, 1,600, or 1,800 calories a day without doing any calculations. The calories are broken down for each meal so you know how many calories are represented on each plate of food. (I generally stop there, but if you really need to know how many calories are in each portion of food on your plate, there's a calorie chart at the back of the book.) What's important now is that you pay attention to the actual measured amounts (portion sizes) and variety of food groups at each meal.

You don't have to pick or stick to one calorie level. You can lose weight by staying within a range of calories. Most women can lose weight within a range of 1,400 to 1,800 calories, depending on current weight and activity levels. Many men can lose weight at average calorie levels of 2,000 and more. Obviously if you stay within your chosen calorie range but don't meet your goal of losing a pound a week, you may have to adjust your range. At the same time, however, look at other factors such as how much exercise you get every day. To know how low you can go with respect to calories, take your current weight and multiply it by ten. If you weigh 165 pounds, your daily calorie intake shouldn't drop much below 1,650. Otherwise, your metabolism might start to slow down, you'll burn calories more slowly, and you'll just defeat your own purpose. As you lose weight, you can lower your calorie limit accordingly.

Advice from Losers

"I didn't have any boyfriends in high school because I was fat, and I have to admit, it was a crush on a guy that first motivated me to lose weight. But then I got the guy, dumped him, and continued to lose weight on my own because I loved the way I was starting to look and feel. I lost 60 pounds in 10 months, and I've kept it off. I've never counted calories. I just make very conscious decisions about what I eat. And I still have fun. I eat out, and I drink beer sometimes. I just eat until I'm satisfied, and if I overeat, I just do some extra exercise that week."

—Alexandra S.

Here's what I suggest: Stick pretty close to these sample menus for a few days, adjusting the calorie level within your chosen range. Pay attention to the variety of foods at each meal, the portion size of each type of food, and the total amount of food at each meal and for the entire day. How does this menu compare to the amount of food you typically eat every day at each meal (which you tracked using a food diary, as covered in Chapter 9)? Is it more? Less? About the same? Knowing that this menu represents about 1,500 calories, can you guess how many calories you normally eat in a day?

Menu Sampler

Who says you can't eat cheese-and-cracker snacks in the afternoon or bacon and eggs for breakfast? With a little planning, you can eat any food you want and still stick to a healthy eating plan. The secret is balance.

The key to this plan is flexibility and learning by doing. Following are three simple, balanced, low-fat menus that provide about 1,500 calories each. That's a good place to start, but if you find you're too hungry or losing weight too quickly or you're not able to lose about a pound a week at this calorie level, you'll have to make adjustments. You can adjust these menus up or down calorie-wise, and you can personalize them to suit your own taste and your own eating style, using the simple tips and suggestions below. You can also follow the menus as written. If you need more menu choices, you'll find some in Chapter 21, "Your Menu for Weight Loss."

Use the blank spaces at the right sides of the sample menus to practice making up your own meal plans. Here's how to personalize these menus:

➤ Substitute any foods you like, from similar food groups, in equal amounts. For instance, any meat or fish or meat substitute such as tofu can be substituted for chicken. Picture the size of a small boneless chicken breast and that's the amount of meat you can have in its place. Substitute any one vegetable for another. Ditto for fruit, dairy products, and grains. That will help keep the menus nutritionally balanced as well as calorically balanced.

➤ If you're unsure about substitutions, look up foods in a calorie chart (see Appendix A, "Calorie and Fat Chart for Selected Foods"), and see how they compare. For instance, if you want an English muffin instead of a slice of toast, you'll find that one half an English muffin has about the same number of calories as one slice of bread.

➤ Practice using common sense. If you want dessert with dinner, skip the snacks during the day. If you want to substitute a different grain or starch for rice, substitute an equal amount. If you're not sure about portion sizes, always lean toward a little less.

➤ Have a glass of wine with dinner and these become 1,650-calorie menus. Don't substitute alcohol calories for food calories. Instead, follow a lighter menu the next day.

➤ The first menu shown is for someone who likes to have a couple of snacks during the day. If you're not a snacker, you can incorporate the calories from those snacks into the three main meals.

➤ Low-calorie and reduced-fat foods are used where they're indicated on the menus. Otherwise, the calorie count is calculated on full-calorie, full-fat varieties of food. For instance, on Menu 2, calories were allowed for whole milk in your coffee, in case you're having the bacon-and-eggs-for-breakfast menu at a local coffee shop that doesn't carry skim milk. Obviously, you'll save calories if you substitute a low-calorie food where a full-calorie food is listed.

➤ To increase the calorie level of these menus, add additional foods, rather than increase the portion size of the food you're already eating. For instance, add a banana to a cereal, milk, and juice breakfast rather than have more cereal.

Menu 1

Breakfast	**Breakfast**
1 cup orange juice ¾ cup bran flake cereal ½ cup skim milk	

Mid-Morning Snack	**Mid-Morning Snack**
½ cup low-fat yogurt, any flavor 2 graham crackers	

Lunch	**Lunch**
½ cup canned tuna packed in water 1 tablespoon reduced-fat mayonnaise 2 slices bread, any type 1 large pear	

Afternoon Snack	**Afternoon Snack**
2 crackers 1 ounce cheese	

Dinner	**Dinner**
1 small chicken breast, sautéed in 2 teaspoons olive oil ½ cup rice (cooked without fat) 4 broccoli spears ½ cup cherry tomatoes Fresh spinach or Romaine lettuce leaves 1 tablespoon reduced-fat salad dressing 1 small breadstick	

Menu 2

Breakfast	**Breakfast**
½ cup orange juice 2 fried eggs	

continues

continued

2 slices crisp bacon

1 slice whole wheat bread

1 tablespoon jelly or jam

¼ cup milk

Lunch	Lunch

Ham sandwich made with

2 ounces (2 slices) lean ham

2 slices whole-wheat bread and

2 teaspoons mustard

Lettuce and tomato salad

1 tablespoon low-calorie dressing

1 apple

Dinner	Dinner

6 ounces cod or other fish broiled with

1 teaspoon olive oil

1 small baked potato

¼ cup fat-free sour cream or yogurt

1 cup steamed green beans

1 cup fresh pineapple chunks

Menu 3

Breakfast	Breakfast

½ grapefruit

½ toasted bagel

2 tablespoons jelly or jam

1 cup skim milk

Lunch	Lunch

1 cup black bean soup

1 small corn muffin

Avocado salad made with

¼ avocado

1 chopped tomato

1 cup torn romaine lettuce leaves and	
1 tablespoon reduced-fat ranch dressing	
1 orange	
Afternoon Snack	**Afternoon Snack**
1 cup fruit-flavored low-fat yogurt	
Dinner	**Dinner**
1 cup cooked pasta spirals	
¼ cup marinara sauce	
1 tablespoon grated Parmesan cheese	
1 small slice Italian bread	
Italian-style salad made with	
1 cup raw spinach leaves	
2 ounces cubed reduced-fat mozzarella cheese	
1 roasted red pepper, sliced	

Keeping the Record Straight

Most people who are concerned about their weight own a bathroom scale. I've known some rather obsessive types who own their own medical scales! Weighing yourself once a week is certainly one way to self-monitor and get a measure of your own success. Sometimes weighing-in can give you a much needed push to work a little harder to get to your goal. Just don't be a slave to your scale!

Accurate scales don't lie, but remember that they might not reflect your true weight on any given day. Your weight can vacillate for a variety of reasons including changes in body fluid levels, hormone fluctuations, and the type of food choices you made that day. None of these reasons have anything to do with your true weight. When you weigh yourself

> **No Weigh!**
> Don't be alarmed if the number on your scale occasionally moves up a little instead of moving down, even when you're doing everything you can to lose weight. A certain amount of weight fluctuation is normal from day to day and even within the same day.

➤ Weigh once a week.

➤ Weigh on the same day of the week at the same time of day.

➤ Weigh yourself naked and dry.

You can keep a record of your weekly weight changes on the weight change chart on the following page.

Weight Change Chart

This chart graphs your weight change from week to week so you can keep track of how much weight you lose and also how your weight fluctuates from time to time. Begin by filling in your current weight at "0." When you weigh yourself in a week, go to week number 1 at the bottom of the graph. Then move up the graph until you reach the row for the number that represents your weight change. For instance, if you lost a pound, stop at the –1 row. Put a dot or X in the box there. Do the same every week, and if you like, connect the dots for a better sense of the direction your weight is taking.

+2																
+1																
Starting Weight ___ 0																
–1																
–2																
–3																
–4																
–5																
–10																
–15																
–20																
–25																
–30																
Week	1	2	3	4	5	6	7	8	9	10	11	12	13	14	15	16

Your Incentive Plan

It's hard to break old habits when you're making lifestyle changes that lead to healthier living. You have to come up with new ideas for filling time that you used to spend eating, and you need distractions from your usual routine. Just as you're learning to balance your meals and balance the amount of food you eat with the amount of exercise you do, you can learn to balance the rest of your life. One way to do that is to come up with new, healthier ways of entertaining and rewarding yourself.

What are your incentives for losing weight and getting fit? Think about all the things you want out of life that depend on your good health. Maybe you want to be better at sports. Maybe you want to live to see your granddaughter through college. Think about the incentives in your own life and write them down. You can refer to them on those days when your attitude seems to be, "Why bother?"

Nonfattening Diversions

Here's are some things you can do with yourself instead of eating. Add some ideas of your own to the bottom of the list. When you're tempted to eat out of boredom, loneliness, or frustration, review the list and pick an alternative activity. The more options you have when you look at the list, the more likely you are to find something you want to do as much as eat.

➤ Have a manicure or pedicure.
➤ Set up a fish tank.
➤ Rent a movie.
➤ Take a short train or bus ride.
➤ Sign up for a class: yoga, low-fat cooking, or art history, for example.
➤ Volunteer at a local hospital or community center.
➤ Visit an art gallery.
➤ Attend a makeup demonstration in a department store.
➤ Read a new magazine.
➤ Change a light bulb.
➤ Browse in a bookstore or library.
➤ Set up a budget.
➤ Build a dollhouse or a doghouse.
➤ Call a friend.
➤ Get a massage.
➤ Go to a park.
➤ Buy a bouquet of fresh flowers.
➤ Take a walk anywhere.
➤ _____
➤ _____
➤ _____
➤ _____

A Job Well Done

Your best reward for getting fit is your own good health, of course, and ideally, that is enough incentive to keep you moving toward your long-term goals. But let's face it. We're all human here, and once in a while, we need material rewards. Some of the diversions listed, such as a massage or a bouquet of flowers, might be considered rewards in and of themselves. Come up with a list of things that you will truly find rewarding. You might take yourself to the ballet or buy a hard-cover book. You might get a facial or buy an expensive moisturizer. For many people, the best material reward is buying clothes a size or two smaller.

Advice from Losers

"I'm 5'5", and now I weigh about 120 pounds. Last year I weighed 150 pounds. I got tired of feeling overweight and unhealthy so I just stopped eating so much junk and just started eating more fruits and vegetables. Then I started exercising with aerobic videos. In the summer I play tennis and swim. I gave myself a reward for every five pounds I lost. It could be anything except food. At first it was another exercise video or a book, but then it was always a new, smaller outfit because that was the most meaningful reward of all. I still reward myself just because I did it!"

—Amy C.

The Least You Need to Know

➤ You need a minimum number of calories every day just to stay healthy. No matter how much weight you want to lose, don't go below 1,200 calories a day without consulting a physician or a registered dietitian. A good rule of thumb is to multiply your current weight by ten and use that figure as your minimum calorie guideline.

➤ It's more sensible to give yourself a calorie range, rather than a single-figure calorie limit.

➤ Once you know what a reasonable serving size looks like, you won't have to worry about the amount of calories in every piece food you eat.

➤ When you eat a balanced diet, you can eat any food you like.

➤ Nonfattening rewards and diversions are important when you're making lifestyle changes to manage your weight.

Part 4
Nutrition 101

Because everybody eats, everybody has an opinion about food and nutrition. Some people raise their eyebrows in disbelief when I say I eat meat. Some mothers look dubious when I say that milk is good for their kids or that sugar might not be responsible for their wild behavior. I've had weight lifters get angry when I suggest they might be wasting money on some of the supplements they're taking. All of these people believe they're making the right nutritional decisions for themselves and their families. On the other end of the spectrum is Morris, my accountant of many years, who makes a very big show out of eating fried pork rinds in front of me. He knows he's making a questionable choice, and he's proud of it!

Consider this part of the book a free course in basic nutrition. In these chapters, you'll learn how your body uses nutrients from the food you eat. You'll also learn how the foods you choose affect your body and help it run more efficiently, or less efficiently, depending on those choices. If you want to find out which foods are the nutritional superstars and which ones barely make the grade, keep turning the pages. After you read this part, you'll be able to make your own decisions about which foods to include often in your diet and which ones to keep to a minimum.

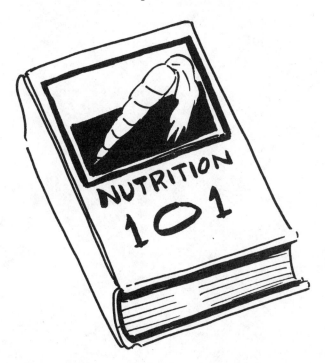

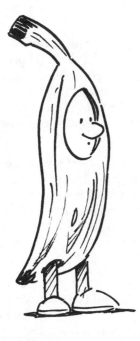

Chapter 11

You Are What You Eat

In This Chapter

➤ What it means to have a metabolism

➤ Calories, calories, and more calories

➤ A course on carbohydrates

➤ A protein primer

➤ Figuring out fat

In self-help circles, motivational leaders like to say you're *not* what you eat. What they mean is, you can't judge yourself by what you eat. It's true. You're not a big fat chunk of cheesecake. That's just a delicious dessert you love to eat. You *are* a body full of protein, carbohydrates, fats, vitamins, minerals, and water. (Not unlike cheesecake.) In that respect, you are very much what you eat.

In this chapter, you'll learn all about energy metabolism, how your body handles calories from different types of foods, and how the different foods you eat affect your weight and your well-being.

Understanding Your Metabolism

You have a metabolism like no one else's. It's unique to you. Your resting, or basal, metabolism is the amount of energy you need to keep your body parts working properly and to maintain a normal body temperature. Beyond that is the energy you use to digest food and absorb nutrients. The technical name for that is the thermic effect of feeding. Last but not least is the thermic effect of activity. That's any energy you use beyond resting and digesting.

When you figured out the number of calories you need to maintain a healthy weight in Chapter 10, "Ready, Set, Go!" you calculated how much fuel you need for energy metabolism. Energy metabolism is the chemical reactions in your body that convert the food you eat into the fuel your body uses for energy. It's not an easy job, but it's one that you want your body to be good at!

No Weigh!
It doesn't take more calories to digest an apple, or any other food, for that matter, than the food itself contains. Although you do burn calories digesting and absorbing food as you eat it, you can't count on that aspect of metabolism to help you control your weight.

Food consists of three basic nutrients that your body can use for energy: carbohydrates, protein, and fat. Each of those nutrients is further broken down into small parts that can be absorbed into your body. That's when energy metabolism begins. Each of the energy nutrients is metabolized differently. Carbohydrates are immediately used to make energy. If you eat more carbohydrates than you need to make energy, some are stored in your liver and muscle and some are converted to body fat. Protein is used to make body protein and is rarely used for energy unless you don't eat enough carbohydrates. Protein that isn't excreted also gets converted to fat. Then there's fat itself, which either is used for energy or is directly stored as body fat.

NutriTip
Once you become an adult, your metabolism slows down and the rate at which you burn calories drops by about two percent every ten years. If you're still eating the same amount of food at age 40 that you were at 20 and not exercising more, you could easily start putting on about 10 pounds a year.

Many factors such as hormones, body temperature, and air temperature affect your body's metabolism and help determine how well you burn calories. Other factors include:

➤ **Body composition.** Muscle is more metabolically active (burns more calories) than fat.

➤ **Age.** Your metabolic rate slows down as you get older. One reason is because you lose muscle mass as you age.

➤ **Gender.** Because women have more fat and less muscle than men, their resting metabolic rates are usually about ten percent lower than those of men who are the same age, height, and weight.

➤ **Physical condition.** When you're in good physical shape from exercise or a job that requires a lot of physical activity, you have more muscle than someone who is more sedentary. As a result, you have a higher metabolic rate.

You can boost your metabolism to burn calories faster than you normally do. The key is exercise. How high you can actually raise your metabolism and what effect the rise will have on your weight depends on many individual things such as your lean body mass and how many calories you consume.

What Is a Calorie Anyway?

Technically speaking, there are no calories in your food. A calorie isn't a "thing." It isn't something you can see, even under a microscope. A calorie is a measurement, like a gram or a pound or a light-year. Calories measure the amount of energy a food supplies to your body. How many calories are in a particular food depends on how much carbohydrate, protein, or fat the food contains:

➤ A gram of carbohydrates provides four calories of energy.

➤ A gram of protein provides four calories of energy.

➤ A gram of fat provides nine calories of energy.

NutriTip
A gram is a metric measurement of weight. When you compare a gram of carbohydrate to a gram of fat, you're comparing equal amounts, by weight, of two different nutrients. It's like comparing a pound of lettuce to a pound of butter, only the amounts are much smaller. A teaspoon of salt, for instance, weighs five grams.

A gram of alcohol, which isn't considered a food because it contains no nutrients, provides seven calories of energy.

When you read the Nutrition Facts label on food packages, you'll see that most foods contain a combination of carbohydrate, protein, or fat. For example, a cup of low-fat (1 percent) milk contains approximately 12 grams of carbohydrate, 8 grams of protein, and 3 grams of fat. Here's how that converts to calories:

12 grams carbohydrate × 4 calories/gram	= 48 calories
8 grams protein × 4 calories/gram	= 32 calories
3 grams fat × 9 calories/gram	= 27 calories
Total calories	107 calories

It helps to know a little diet math so that, for instance, if you want to be sure you're getting only 25 percent of your calories from fat, you'll know how to convert that percentage into actual calories and grams. For example, if your calories total about 1,600 a day, multiply 1,600 by 25 percent (0.25):

$$1,600 \times 0.25 = 400 \text{ calories}$$

400 calories divided by 9 calories/gram = 44.4 grams of fat

Your fat limit at 1,600 calories is 44 grams.

All About Carbohydrates

Carbohydrates are your best source of physical and mental energy. That's one reason why 55–60 percent of your daily calories should come from carbohydrates. We get energy from two types of carbohydrate: simple and complex. When you eat a food rich in either simple or complex carbohydrates, your body breaks down the carbs into a sugar known as glucose. Glucose is a superstar among sugars. When people talk about their blood sugar, they're talking about glucose. Glucose is the only sugar your brain can use as fuel. Glucose is also the sugar that gets stored in your muscles as reserved energy. It's also the sugar that turns into fat if you eat way too much of it.

No Weigh!
No type of sugar is better for you or contains significantly more nutrients than another. Sugar by any other name, whether it's honey, molasses, maple syrup, or turbinado, is still sugar. Only your taste buds know the difference!

Simple carbohydrates are smaller and more easily converted to glucose, so they move more quickly into your bloodstream. Complex carbohydrates take a little more time to break down into glucose and move more slowly into your body, so they don't increase your blood sugar as rapidly. That's especially important to people who have diabetes, hyperglycemia, and other medical problems that affect blood sugar regulation.

It's So Simple!

Chemically speaking, the difference between simple carbs and complex carbs is that simple carbs, also known as simple sugars or single sugars, are less complicated. They arrive in your body as single sugar units that are quickly absorbed into your blood. Foods high in simple carbohydrates include:

➤ White and brown sugars

➤ Honey, molasses, corn syrup, and maple syrup

➤ Candies, cookies, and pastries

➤ Sweetened breakfast cereals

➤ Non-diet soft drinks and sodas

➤ Fruit and fruit juices

Nutritionists don't push simple sugars. You won't hear us recommending candy bars as the mainstay of a healthful diet. That's because most simple sugars add nothing more than calories to your diet. No vitamins, no minerals, no fiber. None of the good stuff. That's why foods high in simple sugars are called "empty-calorie" foods. Fruit is different. A piece of fruit contains plenty of simple sugars, but it also contributes valuable nutrients to your diet, and that's why it's not in the same category as, say, gumdrops.

That doesn't mean nutritionists don't eat gumdrops or pour maple syrup on their pancakes. There's absolutely nothing wrong with eating *some* foods that are high in simple sugars or using them to sweeten other foods. However, it can become a health problem if you're eating cookies, cakes, and other sweets instead of more healthful foods or eating so many desserts and sweet snacks in addition to other foods that you're gaining weight from the extra calories.

It Gets Complex

When simple carbs hook up to one another, they become complex. Complex carbs are the heroes of the carbohydrates world because, in addition to energy-yielding sugar, foods high in complex carbohydrates are also high in important vitamins, minerals, and fiber. Foods rich in complex carbohydrates include:

➤ Grain foods such as flour, pasta, rice, bread, and cereal

➤ Corn, peas, winter squash, and other starchy vegetables

➤ Potatoes and other starchy root vegetables

➤ Legumes such as black beans, kidney beans, lentils, and split peas

Faking It

Whether you use artificial or low-calorie sweeteners is a matter of personal choice. I know people who drink diet sodas but wouldn't dream of using anything other than real sugar in their desserts. Just remember that, like sugar, artificial sweeteners are best used in small measure. Here's the scoop on the fake stuff:

➤ Aspartame, better known as Equal or NutraSweet, has the same 4 calories per gram as sugar, but it's about 200 times sweeter so a little bit goes a long, long way. Commercially, it's used in diet soft drinks, yogurts, fruit spreads, syrups, frozen desserts, and candies, to name just a few products. You can also use aspartame as a tabletop sweetener. People with a rare disease known as phenylketonuria (PKU) cannot use aspartame or any product made with aspartame because this

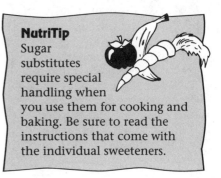

NutriTip
Sugar substitutes require special handling when you use them for cooking and baking. Be sure to read the instructions that come with the individual sweeteners.

sweetener is made with an amino acid (a protein component) that cannot be metabolized by people with PKU.

➤ Acesulfame Potassium or Acesulfame K, known commercially as Sunette, is another man-made sweetener that's about 200 times sweeter than sugar so it is used only in small amounts. It's available as a tabletop sweetener and can be found in pudding and gelatin mixes, chewing gum, breath mints, dessert toppings, and baked goods. It is sometimes used in combination with aspartame.

➤ Saccharin, the original man-made sugar substitute you probably know as Sweet 'N' Low, is about 100 years old now. Although it's seen its share of controversy, it was a hero in both world wars when sugar was scarce and has been a godsend to many people with diabetes. Saccharin is still used as a tabletop sweetener, as sugar is, and it's also used commercially in baked goods, chewing gum, soft drinks, candy, canned fruit, and salad dressings.

Protein Profile

We can't talk about protein without talking first about amino acids, also known as the building blocks of protein. Amino acids are chemical compounds found in food (and in our bodies) that hook together and form proteins. There are 20 different amino acids, and they spend most of their time arranging and rearranging themselves into thousands of different proteins that do thousands of different jobs in your body. These are just a few of the many roles amino acids and proteins play:

➤ Growth. Whenever any part of your body is growing, whether it's bone, blood, or skin, there's a protein at work.

➤ Replacement. Every time you wash your face, you wash off skin cells that must be replaced. Every time you brush your hair or clip your fingernails, protein is needed to replace what's lost.

No Weigh!
Don't be fooled into thinking that eating extra protein will give you tremendous triceps. Yes, you need protein to build muscle, but big muscles come from weight-bearing exercise. The energy for that exercise actually comes from eating carbohydrates.

➤ Repair. When you cut yourself, protein forms the mesh that mends your broken skin and holds it together.

➤ Antibodies. These are proteins found in the blood that help protect us against outside invasion from toxins, viruses, allergens, and bacteria.

➤ Enzymes. All the chemical reactions that happen in your body, such as digestion, require enzymes that are made from proteins.

➤ Hormones. Proteins make up some of your body's most important regulating hormones, such as insulin.

Where Protein Comes From

Your body can make many of the amino acids it needs all by itself, from bits and pieces of chemical fragments that are always floating around in your body anyway. However, there are nine amino acids your body either can't make or can't make enough of. Those nine are called essential amino acids, and they must absolutely come from your diet. Not to worry; as long as you eat a varied, well-balanced diet, you'll get all the amino acids you need.

Individual amino acids aren't stored anywhere in your body. They have no place to go. They're constantly used to make new proteins. If your body isn't using loose amino acids to make new proteins, they break down into smaller parts that get flushed or, on occasion, converted into fat or carbohydrates.

Protein for Vegetarians

For a protein to be usable, it must be complete, which means it must contain all nine essential amino acids. For the most part, animal foods contain all of the essential amino acids and provide your body with complete proteins. Proteins from plant foods, such as vegetables, grains, and beans, tend to be missing one or more essential amino acids or don't contain enough to count as complete.

If you don't eat meat or dairy products, don't worry. Even though proteins from plant foods are for the most part incomplete, they can complement one another and form complete proteins. Don't forget, your body is constantly breaking down and rebuilding proteins from the pool of amino acids that runs through your body. As long as you're eating a variety of grains, seeds, nuts, and vegetables throughout each day, complementary amino acids find one another and hook up to become complete.

It's not necessary to eat complementary proteins at the same meal, although it probably helps ensure that you're getting all the amino acids your body needs to build complete proteins. In some cuisines, such as Mexican, it happens naturally. There's no better complement than rice and beans. The combinations most likely to succeed are grains and legumes or legumes and seeds. A good vegetarian cookbook, such as *The Endangered Broccoli Forest* by Mollie Katzen (Ten Speed Press) or Nikki and David Goldbeck's *American Wholefoods Cuisine* (New American Library), can show you how to prepare winning combos such as:

> **NutriTip**
> Soy foods (made from soybeans) can provide vegetarians with protein and other nutrients that nonvegetarians get from meat, milk, and other dairy products. Soy flour, soy cheese, soy milk, tofu, and other soy products are found in all health food stores and in many large supermarkets.

➤ Tofu and mixed vegetables with fried rice

➤ Chinese noodles with peanut sauce and sesame seeds

➤ Pasta soup with beans and vegetables

➤ Lentil soup with macaroni and vegetables

When you think about it, most vegetarian sources of protein are low in fat and that gives them a distinct advantage over many animal foods. The challenge in cooking vegetarian-style foods is to keep them free of too much added fat.

How Much Protein Do You Really Need?

You don't have to worry about how much of each amino acid you need to eat, but we do have the Recommended Dietary Allowances (RDAs) as a guide for total protein. The RDAs for protein for healthy children and adults are listed in Table 11.1.

Table 11.1 Sample Recommended Dietary Allowances for Total Protein

	Age	Protein (Grams)
Children	1–3	16
	4–6	24
	7–10	28
Males	11–14	45
	15–18	59
	19–24	58
	25+	63
Females	11–14	46
	15–18	44
	19–24	46
	25+	50
Pregnant		60
Lactating	First 6 months	65
	Second 6 months	63

Source: Food and Nutrition Board of the National Academy of Sciences/National Research Council, 1989.

If your RDA for protein is 50 grams, you might divide that throughout the day into approximately 10 grams for breakfast, 15 for lunch, and 25 for dinner. To get an idea of how much food you need to eat to get your daily dose of protein, check out Table 11.2.

Table 11.2 Amount of Protein in Common Foods

Food	Amount	Protein (Grams)
Roast beef, lean	4 oz.	31
Hamburger, lean	4 oz.	32
Turkey, light meat, roasted	4 oz.	34
Chicken, breast, roasted	1 avg.	27
Pork chop, lean, broiled	2½ oz.	23
Flounder, baked	4 oz.	27
Tuna, water-packed	3 oz.	22
Shrimp, large	6	18
Tofu	½ cup	10
Black beans	½ cup	8
Yogurt, low-fat plain	1 cup	12
Milk, low-fat (1%)	1 cup	8
Soy milk	1 cup	7
Peanut butter	2 Tbsp.	8
Sunflower seeds	¼ cup	8
Cottage cheese, low-fat (1 percent)	½ cup	14
Mozzarella cheese, part skim	1 oz.	8
Cheddar cheese	1 oz.	7
Bagel, 3½" diameter	1	7
Oatmeal, cooked	1 cup	6
Chocolate pudding	½ cup	4
Whole wheat bread	1 slice	2

Demystifying Fat

Sometimes it seems all anyone ever thinks about is fat. Everywhere I go, people are talking about fat, worrying about fat, and doing everything they can to avoid fat. It's practically a religion for some people. It borders on neurosis for others. If that sounds like you, read this section carefully.

One thing needs to be perfectly clear: You must have *some* fat in your diet. Fat is a nutrient, and if you eat a totally fat-free diet, your health will suffer. If you don't eat a little fat, you won't be able to absorb the fat soluble vitamins (A, D, E, and K). Your brain and nerves will cease to function effectively. Your skin and hair will get drab. Fat does your body a lot of good, but you don't need a lot of it.

Good Fats, Bad Fats

NutriTip
A *little* fat at every meal is a good thing because it can help make you feel fuller after eating. Fat doesn't leave your stomach as quickly as carbohydrate or protein, so it can keep you feeling full a couple of hours after you eat. If there's no fat at all in your meal, you might be hungry an hour later.

Dietitians love to say, "There are no good foods and no bad foods, just too much of any one food." Basically, that's true, but when it comes to fats, some are clearly better than others. The type of fat you eat, as well as the amount, might affect your risk of getting heart disease or even cancer.

The most healthful fats are found in liquid form. Monounsaturated and polyunsaturated fatty acids found in oils such as olive, corn, canola, and safflower help keep your blood cholesterol and fat levels down. Saturated fatty acids found in meats, butter, lard, and other solid fats and also in palm and coconut oils tend to raise cholesterol and fat levels in your blood. Those are the facts. In the bigger picture, eating too much of *any* kind of fat will make you fat and might eventually make you sick.

What's Your Limit?

How much fat you should eat depends on how many calories you consume overall. Most health experts recommend that we get between 20 and 30 percent of our calories from fat. To figure out your fat max, use this formula:

Total calories × 0.30 calories from fat = maximum calories from fat

An example uses 1,800 calories:

1,800 × 0.30 = 540 calories from fat

If you count fat grams, that translates to

540 calories divided by 9 calories/gram of fat = 60 grams of fat

For quick reference, Table 11.3 shows maximum fat grams for different calorie levels.

Table 11.3 Recommended Maximum Fat Intake by Calorie Level

Total Daily Calories	30 Percent Calories	Fat Grams
1,200	360	40
1,500	450	50
1,800	540	60
2,100	630	70
2,300	690	77
2,600	780	87

Although the total amount of fat you eat should amount to less than 30 percent of your total calories, that doesn't mean every single food or recipe must come in under the 30 percent mark. If your diet is basically balanced, the low-fat foods you eat balance out the higher fat foods over the course of a day or two.

Getting Fat from Fat

It's easier to get fat from eating fat than from eating foods high in carbohydrates or protein, especially if you overeat fat. That's because it's so easy for your body to take extra food fat and store it as body fat. It's practically a direct deposit. Converting carbohydrates and protein to fat is a lot more work, and your body actually burns a good number of extra calories in the process. Also, when your body needs energy, carbohydrate is easily released from your liver and muscle cells—unlike fat. Once fat settles into your fat cells, it doesn't want to budge. The big secret to fighting fat is to not let it settle in the first place! When you follow a low-fat diet, you're trying to get enough fat to do the jobs fat needs to do in the body, but not too much left over.

Guru's Corner
"The great thing about reducing fat in your diet to reduce your weight is that you're also reducing your risk for so many chronic diseases. And you only have to cut back on one small group of foods; there are still hundreds of foods you can eat freely."

—Jo-Ann Heslin, M.A., R.D., coauthor of *The Fat Attack Plan* (Simon & Schuster)

Fake Fats

Ever wonder what goes into reduced-fat and fat-free foods to replace the fat that comes out? When some or all of the fat is removed from salad dressings, ice creams, cheeses, and other dairy products and baked goods such cakes and cookies, food manufacturers use fat substitutes made from carbohydrates and proteins. Some fat replacers are even made from altered forms of fat that your body can't absorb. Check the ingredient list to see what's taking the place of fat in the product you're using:

➤ Carbohydrate-based fat substitutes include modified starches, dextrins, cellulose, and gums. When these products are combined with water, they swell up and can be used to thicken foods such as fat-free mayonnaise and salad dressings.

➤ Protein-based fat substitutes, such as Simplesse, are made with protein from skim milk or egg whites. They lend a creamy texture to such foods

No Weigh!
Don't assume that a low-fat food product is also low in calories. That's rarely true. Most fat replacers used by food manufacturers add calories back to food, often in the form of sugars. As often as not, reduced-fat and fat-free foods provide almost as many calories as the original product. Check the Nutrition Facts labels and compare products so you know what you're eating.

as low-fat ice cream and frozen yogurt. They're also used to improve the texture and appearance of reduced-fat cheeses.

➤ Fat-based substitutes such as Olean (Olestra) and Salatrim are made from chemically altered fatty acids. Olestra, which is used in fried snack foods, adds no calories to food because it passes through your body without being absorbed. Salatrim, found in baked goods, dairy products, and chocolate chips, provides only five calories per gram (compared to fat's nine calories per gram) because it is only partially absorbed by your body.

The Least You Need to Know

➤ Many factors, including your age, body composition, and physical condition, affect the speed of your metabolism.

➤ A calorie is a measurement of the amount of energy a food provides. A gram of carbohydrate provides four calories of energy. A gram of protein also provides four calories. A gram of fat provides nine calories of energy.

➤ Carbohydrates are your body's best source of energy.

➤ Protein is important for growth and repair of all your body tissues. Protein is also the main ingredient in the hormones, enzymes, and antibodies that keep your body functioning.

➤ Even as you're trying to cut fat from your diet, keep in mind that fat is a nutrient, and you do need a little of it to stay healthy.

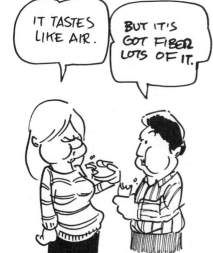

Chapter 12

Non-Caloric Nutrition

In This Chapter

➤ Roughing it up with fiber

➤ Why water is so important in your diet

➤ The many vital roles of vitamins and minerals

➤ What are those phytochemicals doing in your food?

My first meeting with Alex went something like this: In walked a good-looking, 38-year-old guy with a paper bag in his hand. He sat down and told me that every morning, about an hour after he gets out of bed, he gets a bad stomach ache. When I asked him what he did for that first hour after getting up, he opened up his paper bag, took out 16 bottles of dietary supplements and said "I sit at the table, have a few cups of coffee, and take these pills." No wonder he got stomach aches!

The funny thing about Alex was that when I suggested he didn't really need to take any of the supplements, he was relieved. "I'm really glad to hear that," he said. "Because I hate taking all those pills." Like many people, Alex wanted to be healthy and he read a lot of information about vitamins and minerals and other dietary supplements. He thought popping pills was something he was *supposed* to do. It never occurred to him that good nutrition doesn't come from a capsule.

This chapter gives you so many good reasons to eat a balanced diet with a wide variety of foods, especially fresh fruits and vegetables, you'll probably close the book and rush right out to your local greenmarket or supermarket produce department. At least, I hope you will!

You Can't Go Wrong with Roughage

> **NutriTip**
> If you eat a lot of fiber-rich foods, you're eating foods that are naturally low in fat. High-fiber foods, especially starches and grains, are bulky and take time to digest, so you feel fully satisfied after you eat them. When you feel full, you're not as tempted to overeat or start searching for snacks so soon after a meal.

Fiber is a carbohydrate found only in plant foods such as grains, fruits, and vegetables. What makes fiber unique among carbs is that it can't be digested. It passes through your body unchanged. You eat it and excrete it. That's all. So why eat it?

Believe it or not, fiber is just as important to good health as any nutrient you can name. It keeps your digestive system healthy by preventing constipation. It can lower your cholesterol, help control your blood sugar, and soothe the symptoms of irritable bowel syndrome or spastic colon. Some research even suggests that fiber helps fight certain types of cancer. Not bad for a non-nutrient!

All foods that are high in fiber contain two different types of fiber: soluble and insoluble. If you eat a lot of different high-fiber foods, you get plenty of both.

Insoluble Fiber

What your great-grandmother called roughage was really insoluble fiber. Insoluble means that this type of fiber doesn't dissolve in water or body fluids. That's why it's able to help move food right on through your system. Foods that are rich in insoluble fiber help keep you "regular" and also help you fight off digestive diseases such as diverticulosis and colon cancer. Some good examples of foods high in insoluble fiber are

➤ Wheat bran and bran cereals

➤ Bulgur (cracked wheat)

➤ Whole grain breads and other baked goods

➤ Legumes

➤ Vegetables

➤ Fruit

Soluble Fiber

Remember oat bran? Talk about a famous fiber! Most people didn't even know there were two kinds of fiber until scientists discovered that the soluble fiber in oat bran can reduce cholesterol levels.

Soluble means that this type of fiber dissolves in liquids. When mixed with water or body fluids, soluble fiber forms a gel. In your digestive tract, that gel helps to regulate the absorption of both carbohydrate and fats. That's good news for your blood levels of sugar and cholesterol. These are some of the best food sources of soluble fiber:

➤ Legumes

➤ Oats

➤ Barley

➤ Fruit

How Much Fiber Is Enough?

That's a very personal question. In other words, it depends on the person. The recommended range is 20 to 35 grams a day. Although 35 grams of fiber might be necessary to keep things moving for some people, it can be an explosive amount for others, if you know what I mean. Tread carefully when you enter the world of fiber. Too little, and your digestive system can get all blocked up. Too much, and you can end up with painful cramping, bloating, and diarrhea. You can see why it's important to find a happy medium.

If you think you can use more fiber in your diet, add it gradually over a period of a few weeks, and be sure to drink plenty of water to help the extra fiber move through your body. Fiber soaks up fluids like a sponge, and if there isn't enough extra water to move every-thing through, you'll find yourself uncomfortably jammed up. Table 12.1 tells you how much fiber you'll find in a single serving of common foods.

Guru's Corner
"Some high-fiber foods are gas-forming and can cause stomach bloating if you eat too much at once. That's the last thing you want when you're trying to feel lean and fit! If you don't combine too many high-fiber foods at one meal, you should be okay. But a raw-vegetable salad with bean chili could spell disaster if you're not used to that much fiber."

—Regina Ragone, M.S., R.D., weight management counselor

Table 12.1 Fiber in Foods

Food	Amount	Fiber (Grams)
Bran flakes	$3/4$ cup	5.0
Barley, cooked	$1/2$ cup	4.4
Shredded wheat	$3/4$ cup	4.0
Wheat bran, raw	$3/4$ cup	2.0
Oat bran, raw	$1/3$ cup	4.8
Macaroni, cooked	1 cup	2.5

continues

Table 12.1   Continued

Food	Amount	Fiber (Grams)
Bread, whole wheat	2 slices	3.2
Kidney beans, cooked	$^1/_2$ cup	6.6
Broccoli, cooked	1 cup	5.4
Carrot, raw	1 medium	2.1
Potato, baked	1 medium	4.9
Strawberries	1 cup	3.9
Apple, unpeeled	1 large	3.6
Apple, peeled	1 large	2.6
Banana	1 medium	2.9
Grapefruit	$^1/_2$	2.5

NutriTip
Water has no calories, of course, which makes it the perfect drink if you're trying to lose weight and don't want to waste precious calories on fluids. Besides keeping you hydrated, water can help you feel full.

Drink Up!

Water is life itself. You might live for weeks without eating any food at all, but you'd die in just a few days if you didn't have water. You need a constant flow of water through your body to keep your blood flowing, your joints moving, your muscles working, and your lungs breathing. Every part of your body contains and needs water, even your bones.

Every day you lose about ten cups of water through perspiration, breathing, excretion, and evaporation. You lose even more in very hot weather or whenever you work up an extended sweat from exercise. To avoid dehydration, you have to get 8 to 12 eight-ounce cups of water back into your body every day to replace what you lose.

Other Watering Holes

The surest way to get enough water is to drink it regularly, straight from a tap or a bottle. A lot of other fluids and many solid foods contain enough water to make a significant contribution. Water from milk, juices, herbal teas, and diet sodas can help you meet your daily quota. Some foods that supply a good gulp of water with every bite include

➤ Apples

➤ Lettuce

➤ Cucumbers

➤ Grapefruits

➤ Tomatoes

➤ Watermelon

➤ Yogurt

When More Is Better

It's practically impossible to overdose on water, so drink a lot of it. It's better to drink a little more than enough than to risk dehydration. (If you regularly drink more than four or five quarts a day, however, check with your doctor.)

If you eat a diet high in fiber or salt, you might need more than the recommended 8 to 12 cups of water every day. (On the other hand, if your diet is high in watery fruits and vegetables, you might need to drink a little less.) When you exercise, especially in warm weather or if your workout is particularly intense, it's a good idea to drink a glass of water before you start, during your workout, and immediately after. Any time you're exposed to extremely hot or extremely cold weather, you need more water. Flying in an airplane can cause dehydration because the dry, recirculated air on the plane combined with the high altitude causes evaporation of water from your skin. Here are some tips to help you develop a water habit:

No Weigh!
Don't wait until you feel thirsty to drink water. Unfortunately, thirst isn't a good indicator of how much water you need. Some people never feel thirsty at all but still need water. Make it a habit to drink water routinely, even if you don't feel thirsty.

➤ If it doesn't come automatically, ask for water the minute you sit down in a restaurant. Besides helping you meet your water needs, it can take the edge off your appetite.

➤ Whenever you see a water fountain, have a sip.

➤ Carry a water bottle with you wherever you go.

➤ Have a glass of water when you wake up in the morning—before you have your coffee.

➤ If you don't like plain water, add a squeeze of fresh lemon or lime.

➤ When you're at a party, alternate water with other drinks.

Alcoholic beverages and drinks that contain caffeine, such as coffee, tea, caffeinated water, and some soft drinks, act as diuretics and cause you to lose water, so they don't count toward your eight cups a day.

Getting Your Vitamins and Minerals

What vitamins and minerals have in common is that they work together to keep your body functioning properly. You need to include each and every one of them in your diet to stay healthy, but you only need them in small amounts. That's why they're called "micronutrients." Vitamins and minerals don't supply energy to the body, such as carbohydrates, proteins, and fats, but they do help out in the process of converting food to energy. Each vitamin and mineral plays a separate but equal and often interactive role in keeping your body healthy.

Vital Vitamins

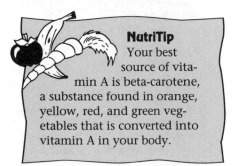

NatriTip
Your best source of vitamin A is beta-carotene, a substance found in orange, yellow, red, and green vegetables that is converted into vitamin A in your body.

There are two categories of vitamins: water soluble and fat soluble. The water solubles include vitamin C and the eight vitamins that make up the B-complex family (B1, B2, B3, B6, B12, folic acid, biotin, and pantothenic acid). The fat solubles include vitamins A, D, E, and K. It doesn't matter whether vitamins are water or fat soluble; you need to get both!

Table 12.2 explains what the different vitamins do for your health and the best food sources of each.

Table 12.2 Where to Get Your Vitamins

Vitamin	Necessary for	Best Food Sources
A	Normal vision, healthy skin, tissue repair, and growth.	Red, yellow, and orange fruits and vegetables such as sweet potatoes, red peppers, cantaloupe, carrots, tomatoes, and green leafy vegetables such as spinach.
B1 Thiamin	Normal function of heart, nerves, muscle, and digestive system.	Lean meat, enriched cereals and baked goods, legumes, and nuts.
B2 Riboflavin	Energy production, healthy immune system and skin.	Low-fat dairy products, lean meats, eggs, and enriched cereals and baked goods.
B3 Niacin	Energy production, healthy skin, reproductive, and digestive systems.	Lean meat, seafood, poultry, legumes, nuts, enriched cereals and baked goods, and leafy green vegetables.
B6	Energy production, red blood cell production, and growth.	Lean meat, seafood, legumes, enriched cereals and baked goods, and leafy green vegetables.
B12	Energy production and red blood cell production.	Lean meat, poultry, seafood, eggs, low-fat dairy products, and tempeh.
Biotin	Fat and protein metabolism and energy production.	Egg yolks; found in small amounts in a wide variety of foods.
Folic acid	Energy production, red blood cell formation, and growth.	Lean meat, seafood, legumes, leafy green vegetables, and whole grains.

Vitamin	Necessary for	Best Food Sources
Pantothenic acid	Carbohydrate, fat, and energy metabolism and growth.	Lean meat, seafood, poultry, legumes, and whole grains.
Vitamin C	Growth, wound healing, disease resistance, and bone and teeth formation.	Citrus fruits, berries, sweet and hot peppers, leafy green vegetables, tomatoes, and potatoes.
Vitamin D	Growth, healthy bones, teeth, and nails, and proper absorption of calcium.	Fortified milk and milk products; vitamin D is also synthesized from sunlight that reaches your skin.
Vitamin E	Protection of cell membranes and nerves.	Vegetable oils, margarine, and avocado.
Vitamin K	Clotting and bone formation.	Green leafy vegetables, broccoli, and dairy products.

Minerals Are a Must

There are least 22 minerals known to be essential for good health. Most are trace minerals, which means we need only tiny, tiny amounts to stay healthy. The trace minerals include iron, zinc, and selenium. Other minerals such as calcium, potassium, and sodium are needed in larger amounts, so they're called major minerals. The majors are no more important to your health than the minors. Table 12.3 gives the scoop on some of the more common minerals.

NutriTip
Lean red meat is a source of iron, but it's also found in non-meat foods such as enriched breads and cereals, legumes, and dried fruit such as prunes and raisins. Your body doesn't absorb as much iron from non-meat sources, but you can help it along by eating foods high in vitamin C at the same time.

Table 12.3 Minerals in Your Diet

Mineral	Necessary for	Best Food Sources
Calcium	Healthy bones, teeth, nails, and muscle and normal heart and nerve function.	Low-fat dairy products such as milk, yogurt, and cheese and leafy green vegetables such as kale and broccoli.
Iron	Healthy red blood cells and prevention of anemia.	Lean red meats, shellfish, legumes, dried fruit, and leafy green vegetables.
Potassium	Balancing body fluids and normal heart rhythm.	Fruits, vegetables, dried fruits, legumes, and low-fat milk.
Selenium	Protects body cells.	Seafood, lean meats, and grains.
Sodium	Regulating body fluids and normal nerve and muscle function.	Almost all foods contain sodium, especially processed foods.
Zinc	Normal appetite and taste, wound healing, and normal growth.	Lean meat, shellfish, wheat germ, and legumes.

What About Supplements?

The more you cut calories, the harder it is to get all the vitamins and minerals you need from your diet. You have to be much more careful about the types of food you eat. If you eat a well-balanced, carefully planned diet, you probably don't need a supplement. If for any reason you're on a very low calorie diet or you can't eat a balanced diet that includes foods from all food groups, however, you might consider taking a multivitamin-mineral supplement.

No Weigh!
No pill can take the place of a well-balanced diet. A vitamin and mineral supplement should do just that: It should *supplement* an otherwise healthful diet. Learn how to choose nutrient-rich foods and then, if you're on a low-calorie diet, ask a doctor or a dietitian if a supplement is necessary.

As with everything else in life, moderation is the key to taking supplements. More isn't better in this case because too much can hurt you. If you choose to take a multivitamin and mineral supplement, pick one that provides no more than 100 percent of the daily value for each nutrient. More than that and you're in danger of overdosing.

Because minerals and fat-soluble vitamins are stored in your body, taking large doses in supplements can actually be toxic to your system. High doses of water-soluble vitamins can also make you sick and in some cases, cause serious damage to your liver, kidney, and nervous systems. Too much of any one vitamin or mineral can interfere with the absorption or metabolism of another. For instance, too much calcium can block iron absorption. You can actually lose precious vitamins and minerals by taking too many of them!

If you're in the market for a multivitamin-mineral supplement, here are a few tips to help you choose what's best for you:

➤ Check the expiration date on the label. Nutrients lose their potency after a certain period of time.

➤ In general, "natural" supplements have no nutritional advantage over synthetic nor do name brands over generic.

➤ Some supplements might interfere with medications, so check with your doctor or pharmacist if necessary.

➤ Avoid supplements that contain any nutrient in a dose higher than the daily value for that particular nutrient.

➤ If you have young children in your home, buy supplements in childproof containers.

These days, vitamins and minerals aren't the only nutrients sold in capsules and pills. A lot of other dietary supplements are crowding the shelves. Most of them can't do what they imply they can do. Most of the claims for these products are scientifically unproven. Some supplements are promoted as vitamins when in fact, they're not. Remember this: If you're healthy, supplements won't make your body work better. If you're not feeling up to par, you need to see a doctor before you diagnose yourself or treat yourself with over-the-counter supplements. Most supplements won't hurt you, but some could. It's a rare person who actually *needs* a dietary supplement, so why waste your money? Some of the more popular and most questionable supplements promoted as energy enhancers, muscle-builders, fat-busters, and weight-loss aids include

> **No Weigh!**
> Don't be tempted to try an herbal or "natural" remedy or weight-loss aid unless you're absolutely sure about the safety of its ingredients.

➤ Amino acids

➤ Bee pollen

➤ Carnitine

➤ Chromium picolinate

➤ Co-enzyme Q10

➤ Creatine phosphate

➤ Laetrile

➤ Pangamic acid

➤ Spirulina (a.k.a. blue-green algae)

Phytochemicals in Your Food

It might sound scary, but the word *phytochemical* simply means plant chemical. It refers to hundreds, if not thousands, of natural substances found in fruits and vegetables. These substances have names such as flavonoid, indole, lycopene, and carotenoid, and they protect the plants themselves from viruses, bacteria, and other toxins. Unlike vitamins and minerals, few phytochemicals have a defined role in the human body as of yet, but scientists are hard at work to determine just how important to your health they may be.

> **NutriTip**
> If you're trying to get your fair share of phyto-chemicals, stick to fresh food sources. Although powdered vegetable extracts are sold as phytochemical supplements, no one knows whether phytochemicals are effective when they're isolated from food, dehydrated, and put into a capsule. No one knows if phytochemicals work when isolated from the food in which they originally come.

The Least You Need to Know

➤ It's important to get just enough fiber in your diet to keep your digestive system healthy and possibly prevent serious disease.

➤ Every day you need to get at least 8 to 12 eight-ounce cups of water from food and fluids to replace what you lose through normal body processes such as perspiration and breathing.

➤ Every vitamin and mineral is as important as the next, and they all work together to regulate different body functions.

➤ Phytochemicals and other as yet unidentified compounds found in fresh fruits and vegetables and other plant foods might be just as important to your health as vitamins and minerals. All the more reason to eat good food!

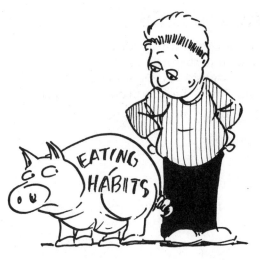

Chapter 13

Take a Look at Your Eating Habits

In This Chapter

➤ A quick hike up the food pyramid

➤ How much food is on your plate?

➤ Using pyramid food groups to balance your diet

➤ Using the pyramid to design a menu for losing weight

This probably isn't the first time you've seen the U.S. Department of Agriculture's Food Guide Pyramid. Have you actually explored it? Okay, I admit it's not as exciting as a trip to Egypt to explore the real pyramids, but it's just as educational. Just like every other tool designed to help you make smarter food choices and maintain a healthy weight, the food pyramid is a guide and a teaching aid. It doesn't represent a rigid set of rules that you have to live by. It's not a weight-loss plan, but it can help you get to a healthy weight. It's more like an outline for healthy eating. You fill it in with the food choices you make.

This chapter takes you step-by-step up the food pyramid, pausing at each level to describe what you'll find there and what it means to you. If your current eating habits don't stack up, you can use the pyramid as a tool to help you reach your healthy weight.

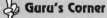

Guru's Corner

"The Food Guide Pyramid is a great tool to use when you're trying to get to a healthy weight because it teaches you how to control your portion sizes and eat a wide enough variety of foods to get all the different nutrients you need."

—Michelle Luhan, M.S., R.D., Nutritionist, New York University Medical Center

Exploring the Pyramid

The food pyramid encourages eating a variety of foods from all five food groups shown in the three lower levels of the pyramid. Each of these groups gives you some, but not all, of the nutrients you need to be healthy. Those groups are

➤ The bread, cereal, rice, and pasta group

➤ The vegetable group

➤ The fruit group

➤ The milk, yogurt, and cheese group

➤ The meat, poultry, fish, dry beans, eggs, and nuts group

The Food Guide Pyramid. Source: United States Department of Agriculture

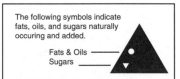

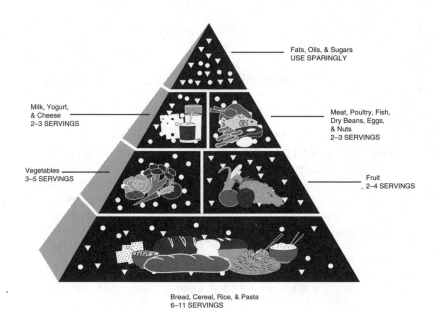

Following are the contributions each food group makes to your diet and the recommended number of servings every day from each group. Let's take a hike up the pyramid and see what these food groups have to offer.

➤ The breads, cereals, rice, and pasta group is at the base of the food guide pyramid. Just as it provides a foundation for the pyramid, this group also represents the foundation of a healthy diet. Foods in this group provide complex carbohydrates for energy, fiber, vitamins, and minerals. The recommended number of servings from this group is 6 to 11 each day.

➤ The vegetable group is on the next tier of the pyramid. If you pick the right vegetables, you'll get a lot of vitamins A and C and folic acid as well as other important vitamins and minerals from this group, not to mention good old reliable fiber. The recommended number of servings from this group is three to five each day.

➤ The fruit group is on the same level as vegetables, and for good reason. Again, if choose your fruits wisely, you'll get a lot of vitamins plus potassium and more fiber. The recommended number of servings from this group is two to four each day.

➤ The milk, yogurt, and cheese group is up close to the top of the pyramid. This is the dairy group, where most of your calcium comes from. You may have noticed by now that as you hike up closer to the tip, you need fewer servings of the foods you find at each level. The recommended number of servings from this group is two for most people and three for teenagers and young adults (under 25) and women who are pregnant or breastfeeding.

➤ The meat, poultry, fish, dry beans, eggs, and nuts group is up there next to the milk group. You get your best protein from foods in this group, plus B vitamins, iron, and zinc. The recommended number of servings from this group is two to three each day, or the equivalent of between five and seven ounces of meat.

➤ The fats, oils, and sweets group at the very tip of the pyramid includes all those "empty calorie foods" that offer very little in the way of good nutrition. You know the ones: fat-filled foods such as salad dressings, oils, creams, butter, margarine and other bread spreads, and sugary foods such as candies, cakes, and soft drinks. Adding too many of these foods to your diet adds a lot of extra calories. These are the foods that can really get in your way when you're trying to lose or maintain your weight. There's no recommended number of servings from this group, just the advice to "use sparingly."

How Much Is Enough?

To know how much food you can eat over the course of a day or at any single meal and not worry about how many calories you're getting, it helps to know standard serving sizes for different foods within each food group. If you've ever followed an exchange system,

141

these serving sizes will, for the most part, look familiar to you. If not, pay close attention to this section. Once you understand the concept of standard serving sizes, designing menus to help you get to a healthy weight becomes a whole lot easier.

What's in a Serving?

Following are the basic recommended serving sizes for foods within each pyramid food group. For the most part, serving sizes in each group are small—probably smaller than you think.

➤ Bread, cereal, rice, and pasta group: One serving from this group provides about 80 calories.

1 slice of any type of bread

$^1/_2$ English muffin

$^1/_2$ small bagel

$^1/_2$ small (6-inch) pita bread

$^1/_2$ hamburger or frankfurter bun

1 small (6-inch) tortilla

1 small ($2^1/_2$ inch diameter) roll or biscuit

1 ounce of ready-to-eat cereal (This amount varies with the type of cereal, from $^1/_4$ cup Grape Nuts to about $^3/_4$ cup bran flakes to about $2^1/_2$ cups puffed cereal.)

$^1/_2$ cup cooked cereal, rice, or pasta

$^1/_4$ cup corn, peas, potatoes, winter squash, legumes, or other starchy vegetable

➤ Vegetable group: One serving from this group provides about 25 calories.

1 cup of raw leafy green vegetables such as spinach, kale, or romaine lettuce

$^1/_2$ cup of any other vegetables, cooked or chopped raw

$^3/_4$ cup of vegetable juice

Starchy vegetables such as corn, peas, potatoes, winter squash, and legumes are counted in the bread group.

➤ Fruit group: One serving from this group provides about 60–80 calories.

1 medium apple, banana, orange, or other fruit

1 cup strawberries, blueberries, or raspberries

$^1/_2$ grapefruit

$^1/_2$ mango

$^1/_2$ cup chopped, cooked, or canned fruit

7 dried apricot halves

10 cherries

10 grapes

3 prunes

2 Tbsp. raisins

³/₄ cup of fruit juice

➤ Meat, poultry, fish, dry beans, eggs, and nuts: One serving from this group provides from about 150–250 calories.

2 to 3 ounces (cooked weight) of lean meat, poultry, or fish

1 to 1¹/₂ cups cooked dry beans (measured after cooking)

1 to 1¹/₂ cups tofu

2 to 3 eggs

Two tablespoons of peanut butter is equivalent to 1 ounce of meat and contributes 200 calories.

➤ Milk, yogurt, and cheese group: One serving from this group provides about 150–200 calories. Reduced-fat and skim milk dairy products may provide fewer calories.

1 cup milk or yogurt

1¹/₂ ounces of natural cheese such as cheddar, blue, brie, feta, gouda, or mozzarella

¹/₂ cup ricotta cheese

¹/₃ cup grated Parmesan or Romano cheese

2 ounces process cheese (2 slices or "singles")

What Does a Serving Look Like?

When you're trying to lose or maintain weight, it's even possible to eat too much of the "good stuff," such as grains and fruit. As you already know, calories count, and even the most nutritious foods can add unwanted calories to your diet. That's why portion control and the concept of serving sizes is such a big deal, especially when your calorie limit is down there around 1,500 or 1,600 a day. The great thing about portion control is that by limiting the amount of each type of food you eat, you get to eat a lot of different foods. Eating many different foods is a good way to be sure you're getting all your nutrients. It's also a good way to prevent boredom!

NutriTip
Remember these visual cues for standard serving sizes:

➤ One serving of meat, poultry, or fish is about the size of a deck of cards or the palm of an average-size hand or a cassette tape case.

➤ A muffin that counts as two bread servings is about the size of a tennis ball.

➤ An ounce of cheese is about the size of a matchbook.

Here are some easy ways to teach yourself what a serving size looks like:

➤ Use a household measuring cup to measure one serving of your favorite cereal into the bowl you normally use. Once you know what that amount of cereal looks like in that particular bowl, you can measure by sight. You only have to remeasure when you switch cereals.

➤ Use the preceding method for a one-time formal measure of foods such as rice, pasta, and vegetables. Take notice of what a $1/2$ cup serving of each of these foods looks like on a dinner plate. That way, whether you're at home, a guest at someone else's table, or out at a restaurant, you'll know how much food you're eating just by looking at it.

Picture This!

The following sketches are life-size representations of actual servings of food from the five different food groups. Compare them to your usual portions of similar foods to see how they measure up.

Muffin (1 small)

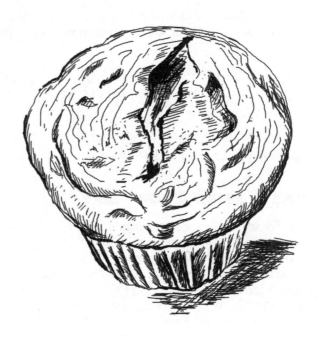

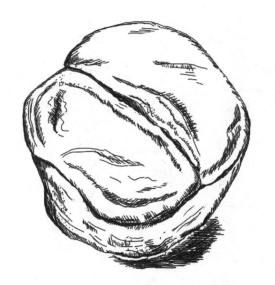

Dinner roll (1 roll)

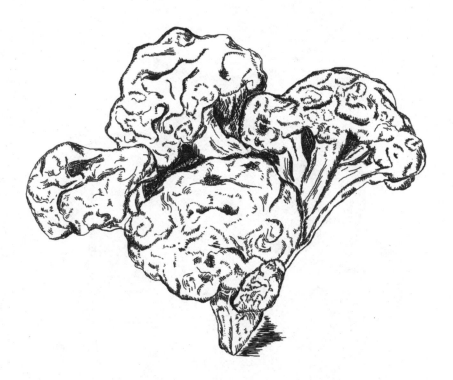

Cauliflower
(¹/₂ cup)

Bagel (¹/₂ bagel)

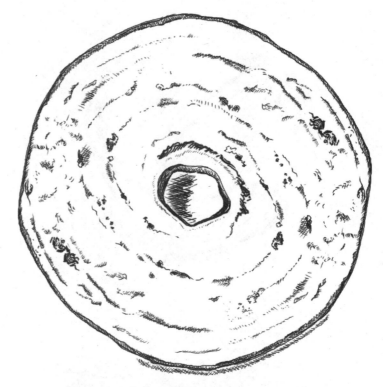

Zucchini (¹/₂ cup)

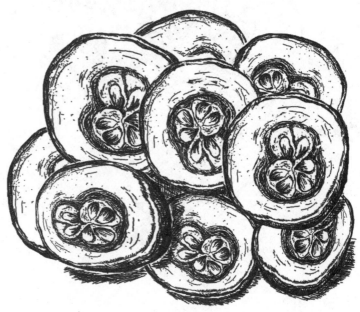

Tofu (¹/₂ cup)

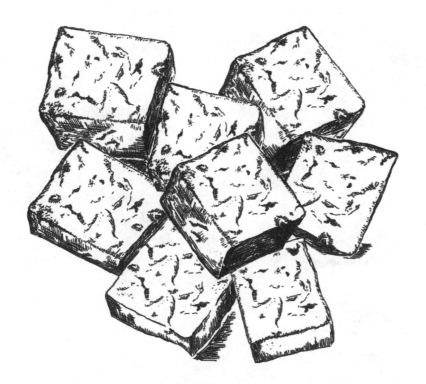

*Ground beef
(3 ounces)*

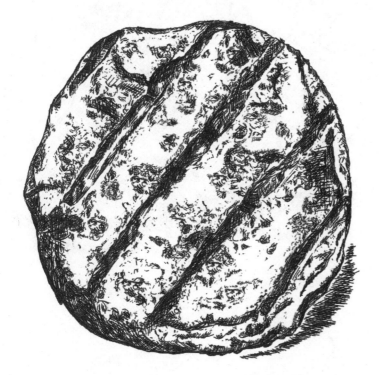

*Roasted chicken
(3 ounces)*

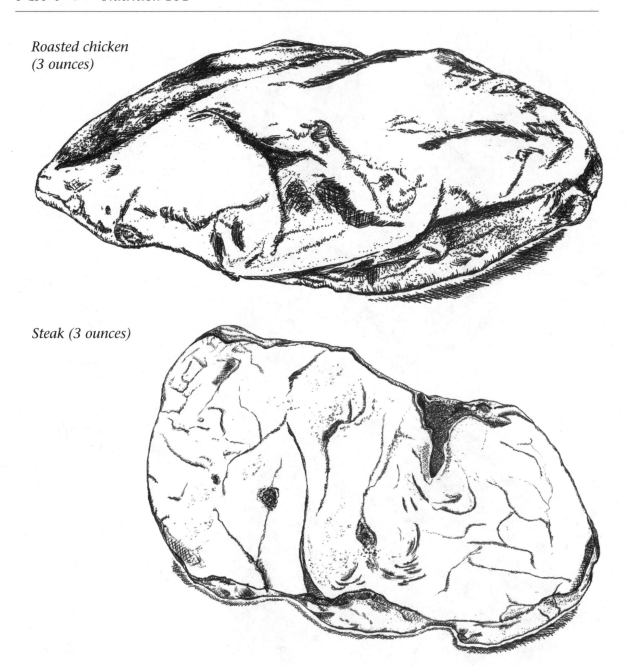

Steak (3 ounces)

Shrimp (3 ounces)

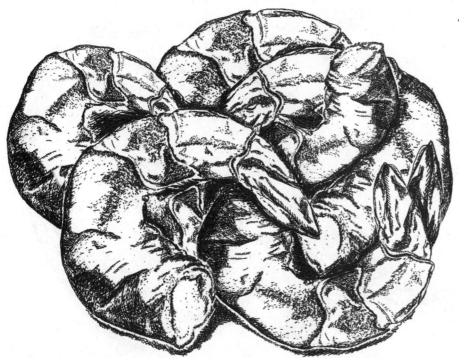

Italian sausage (3 ounces)

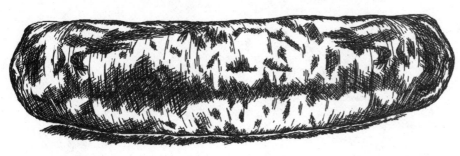

*Pork chop
(3 ounces)*

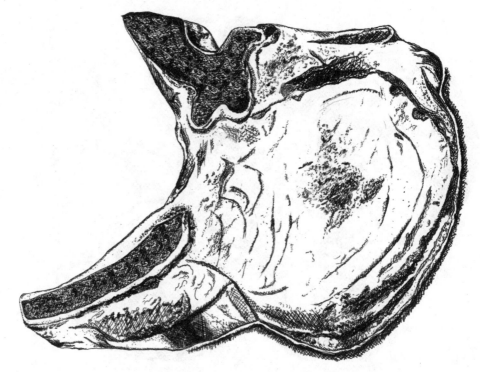

*Sliced cheese
(1 ounce)*

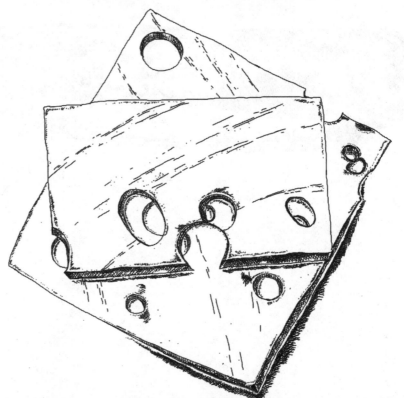

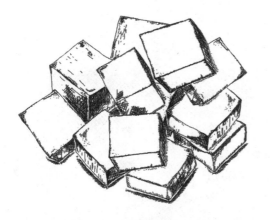

*Diced cheese
(1 ounce)*

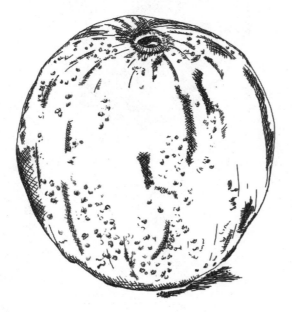

Orange (1 medium)

Apple (1 medium)

*Banana
(1 medium)*

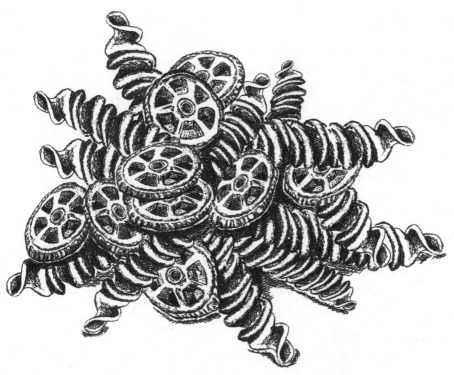

Pasta (¹/₂ cup)

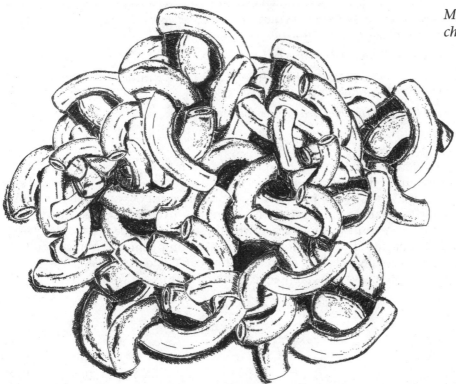

Macaroni and cheese (1 cup)

Balancing Your Meals

The food pyramid is another tool that can help you plan a day's worth of balanced, calorie-controlled meals without actually counting calories. Instead, you can develop menus by choosing a certain number of servings from each of the different food groups. The pyramid shows a range of servings in each group. The number of servings you choose depends on how many calories you need for the day and how active you are. Table 13.1 tells you how many servings you can have from each group for different calorie levels. The number of servings allotted for each calorie level assumes you're making low-fat and lean food choices from each group and not dipping too often into the fats, oils, and sweets group. Obviously, if your calorie count falls above, below, or in between these levels, you'll have to adjust your number of servings.

Table 13.1 Number of Servings by Calorie Level

Approximate calorie level	1,600	2,200	2,800
Bread group servings	6	9	11
Vegetable group servings	3	4	5
Fruit group servings	2	3	4
Milk group servings	2–3*	2–3*	2–3*
Meat group servings	2, for a total of 5 ounces	2, for a total of 6 ounces	3, for a total of 7 ounces

Women who are pregnant or breastfeeding, teenagers, and young adults up to age 24 need at least three servings from the milk group to meet their calcium needs.

A 1,600 calorie diet is recommended for women and older adults.

A 2,200 calorie diet is recommended for children, teenage girls, active women, and sedentary men. Women who are pregnant or breastfeeding may need more calories.

A 2,800 calorie diet is recommended for teenage boys and active men.

Source: USDA, 1992.

Once you know how many servings you can have from each food group, you can divide those servings throughout the day, depending on how you like to eat. For instance, if you have a sausage and egg sandwich for breakfast, you may use most of your protein servings in the morning. Try to balance your meals with a serving or two from at least three different food groups at each meal and at least two different groups for snacks. Following are some examples of balanced, 1,600-calorie menus based on pyramid servings. You'll see that they're not always perfect. Perfection isn't the goal. Good eating is! These samples include fill-in blanks so you can practice pyramid eating on your own.

Pyramid Menu 1: 1,600 Calories	
Breakfast	**Breakfast**
1 English muffin	
2 fried eggs	
1 small glass grapefruit juice	
Pyramid servings: 2 bread group, 1 meat group, 1 fruit group	Pyramid servings:
Lunch	**Lunch**
2 slices whole wheat bread	
2 slices cheddar cheese	
¹/₂ tomato, sliced	
Romaine lettuce	
Pyramid servings: 2 bread group, 2 dairy group, 1 vegetable group	Pyramid servings:
Snack	**Snack**
1 cup low-fat yogurt with	
1 cup strawberries	
Pyramid servings: 1 dairy group, 1 fruit group	Pyramid servings:
Dinner	**Dinner**
Spinach and mushroom salad with low-fat dressing	
1 flour tortilla	
1 cup black beans	
¹/₂ cup cooked white rice	
¹/₂ cup fresh tomato salsa	
Pyramid servings: 2 bread group, 1 meat group, 2 vegetable group	Pyramid servings:

Pyramid Menu 2: 1,600 Calories	
Breakfast	**Breakfast**
1 bowl bran flake cereal	
$^1/_2$ cup low-fat milk	
1 medium banana	
Pyramid servings: 1 bread group, $^1/_2$ milk group, 1 fruit group	Pyramid servings:
Lunch	**Lunch**
2 cups spinach and grated carrot salad topped with	
$1^1/_2$ cups three-bean salad and	
1 breadstick	
1 pear	
Pyramid servings: 1 bread group, 1 meat group, 2 vegetable group, 1 fruit group	Pyramid servings:
Snack	**Snack**
1 cup vanilla pudding*	
2 graham crackers*	
Pyramid servings: 1 bread group, 1 milk group (*Dessert or snack foods can occasionally be included in your plan. Match them to their closest food group.)	Pyramid servings:
Dinner	**Dinner**
Turkey parmesan made with: 3 ounces roast turkey breast	
$^1/_2$ ounce shredded mozzarella cheese	
2 Tbsp. grated Parmesan cheese	
$1^1/_2$ cups cooked pasta	
$^1/_4$ cup marinara sauce	
$^1/_2$ cup steamed broccoli	
Pyramid servings: 1 meat group, 1 milk group, 3 bread group, 1 vegetable group	Pyramid servings:

Putting the Pyramid into Practice

If a typical plate of food at your house still has more meat on it than anything else and your idea of a salad is a chunk of iceberg dripping with creamy Italian, then your diet probably needs a vigorous overhaul. But if on an average day you eat a variety of different foods from different food groups, and the emphasis in your diet is more on carbohydrates than protein and fat, you might just need a little more practice at portion control.

You can use the following Pyramid Menu Plan (photocopy it to make as many copies as you need) as a type of food diary to see how your current diet stacks up against the pyramid. You can also use them as menu planners and incorporate the pyramid plan into your own healthy weight plan. Fill in your total number of servings for each group at the type, and then fill in the number of servings used at each meal, next to the food itself.

Pyramid Menu Plan

Total Daily: ____ Bread group servings   ____ Milk group servings
              ____ Vegetables group servings ____ Meat group servings
              ____ Fruit group servings

Servings	Food
Breakfast	
____	Bread _____
____	Vegetable _____
____	Fruit _____
____	Milk _____
____	Meat _____
Lunch	
____	Bread _____
____	Vegetable _____
____	Fruit _____
____	Milk _____
____	Meat _____
Dinner	
____	Bread _____
____	Vegetable _____
____	Fruit _____
____	Milk _____
____	Meat _____
Snack	
____	_____

The Least You Need to Know

➤ The Food Guide Pyramid is a tool that can help you learn how to plan nutritionally balanced, portion-controlled meals as part of a healthy weight plan.

➤ Each of the five food groups represented on the pyramid contributes some, but not all, of the nutrients you need to stay healthy.

➤ Once you understand what standard serving sizes of different foods look like, you'll know how to control the amount of food you eat wherever you go.

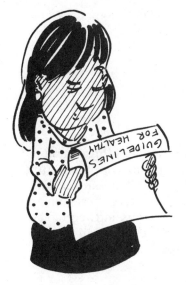

Chapter 14

Guidelines for Healthy Living

In This Chapter

➤ Putting variety in your diet

➤ Balancing food and physical activity

➤ Grains, fruits, and vegetables: Are you getting enough?

➤ A low-fat diet is still the best diet

➤ How sweet it is!

➤ Shaking your salt habit

➤ How alcohol fits into a healthy diet

The U.S. Departments of Agriculture and Health and Human Services developed the *Dietary Guidelines for Americans* so we know how to eat to stay healthy. These are the guidelines:

➤ Eat a variety of foods.

➤ Balance the food you eat with physical activity to maintain or improve your weight.

➤ Choose a diet with plenty of grain products, vegetables, and fruits.

➤ Choose a diet low in fat, saturated fat, and cholesterol.

➤ Choose a diet moderate in sugars.

➤ Choose a diet moderate in salt and sodium.

➤ If you drink alcoholic beverages, do so in moderation.

This chapter shows you how to use these guidelines to choose foods and build eating habits that will help you get to a healthy weight and stay there.

Eat a Wide Variety of Foods

Before there was a food pyramid, there were four food groups: meat, dairy, bread, and fruits and vegetables. Now there are five food groups because the pyramid separated fruits and vegetables into two groups. Foods that are grouped together contribute similar nutrients to your diet. For example, many dairy products are good sources of calcium and vitamin D. The meat group supplies protein, iron, and B vitamins. Fruits and vegetables are great sources of vitamins C and A. The only way to be sure you're getting all the nutrients you need is to eat a variety of foods from all five groups. That's especially important when you're limiting calories to try to lose weight.

NutriTip
Some foods, such as sweet potatoes, spinach, broccoli, cantaloupe, and kiwi, are nutritional superstars. They supply a day's worth of at least one vitamin and a significant amount of others in just a single serving.

It's just as important to eat a variety of foods *within* each food group as it is to choose foods from all five groups. That's because even within each group, different foods supply different nutrients. Fruit is a great source of vitamins. Although some fruits, such as oranges, grapefruits and other citrus, are excellent sources of vitamin C, others, such as cantaloupe, mangoes, and apricots, are also great sources of vitamin A. Some fruits, such as pears, are high in fiber but not particularly high in vitamins or minerals.

Some foods are especially rich in a particular nutrient and some even supply more than an entire day's worth of a nutrient in just one serving. Table 14.1 lists some of the best sources of selected vitamins and minerals we have in our food supply. Compare the nutrient value of these foods to the Daily Value (the government recommendation based on average needs of men and women of all ages) for each nutrient, and you'll see why certain foods are considered especially healthful. If you include a variety of these foods in your diet, you're bound to get all the nutrients you need at almost any calorie level.

Table 14.1 Foods That Are Good Sources of Vitamins and Minerals

Vitamin A
Daily Value: 1,000 retinol equivalents (RE)

1 baked sweet potato	2,486 RE
1 raw carrot	2,024 RE

1 cup cooked spinach	1,474 RE
1 cup mashed butternut squash	1,435 RE
¹/₂ cantaloupe	860 RE
¹/₂ mango	400 RE
1 cup cooked broccoli	210 RE

Vitamin C
Daily Value: 60 milligrams (mg)

1 kiwi	138 mg
1 cup cooked broccoli	110 mg
¹/₂ cantaloupe	110 mg
¹/₂ papaya	98 mg
1 cup cooked Brussels sprouts	95 mg
1 cup fresh strawberries	80 mg
1 cup cooked cauliflower	70 mg
1 orange	70 mg
1 baked potato with skin	26 mg
¹/₂ cup chopped fresh parsley	25 mg

Vitamin E
Daily Value: 8 mg to 10 mg

2 tbsp. sunflower seeds	9 mg
1 tbsp. sunflower oil	7 mg
1 tbsp. safflower oil	5 mg
1 tbsp. Canola	3 mg
1 tbsp. corn oil	3 mg
3 oz. cooked shrimp	3 mg
¹/₂ avocado	2 mg
1 oz. mixed nuts	2 mg
2 tbsp. peanut butter	2 mg
3 oz. cooked salmon	2 mg

Folic Acid
Daily Value: 400 micrograms (mcg)

1 cup cooked spinach	260 mcg
2 cups raw spinach	220 mcg
¹/₂ cup cooked lentils	179 mcg
1 cup cooked asparagus	170 mcg
¹/₂ cup cooked black beans	127 mcg
1 cup cooked beets	80 mcg

continues

Table 14.1   Continued

1 cup cooked broccoli	80 mcg
2 tbsp. wheat germ	35 mcg

Calcium
Daily Value: 1,000 mg

1 cup low-fat plain yogurt	413 mg
1/2 cup part-skim ricotta	335 mg
1 cup 1% low-fat milk	300 mg
3 oz. sardines	300 mg
1 oz. cheddar cheese	205 mg
1 cup cooked kale	180 mg
3 oz. canned salmon	150 mg
1 oz. 1% low-fat cottage cheese	137 mg
1 cup cooked broccoli	80 mg

Iron
Daily Value: 18 mg

1 cup tofu	14 mg
1 cup cooked lentils	7 mg
4 oz. lean beef sirloin	4 mg
1 cup cooked white beans	4 mg
1 baked potato	3 mg
1 cup prune juice	3 mg
3 oz. cooked shrimp	3 mg
1 cup split pea soup	2 mg

Finding Balance

Whenever there's a shift in the balance between how much food you eat and how much exercise you do, your weight will start to move up or down. If your work schedule changes and you suddenly have no time to get to the gym, your balance shifts, and eventually, you'll start to feel a bit weightier unless you also cut back on the amount of food you eat. When you're trying to lose weight, you're intentionally trying to shift the balance so that you use more calories than you consume by eating less and exercising more. Once you've reached your goal weight, you'll try to maintain the balance of food and activity that keeps you at that weight.

If you're like most people, you spend most of your day sitting, or perhaps standing, and not doing much moving. When you come home, it's more of the same. To balance the calories you consume from food and drinks every day, you have to design an activity plan that matches your food plan. You'll read all about exercise in Part 5, "Exercise 101," but right now is a good time to start thinking about different ways you can increase your activity on most, if not all, days of the week. The following are some tips if you're considering exercising for the first time:

➤ Only choose exercises and activities that you enjoy. If you don't like running or tennis or stair-masters, go dancing!

➤ Try to exercise with other people sometimes so you'll have more fun.

➤ Find a physical activity that's also a hobby, such as hiking into the woods to identify mushrooms or insects.

➤ Change your activity from time to time to keep exercise fresh.

NutriTip
Balance is something you have to strive for and work toward. It doesn't just come naturally to most people. It doesn't matter whether you're talking about your diet or your life. You have to learn what it takes to find your own balance. Obviously, it's more than having the right mix of foods on your plate.

Age is no excuse for getting out of shape. If you're active now, try to maintain the same level of exercise as you get older. If you're not active, start slow and build up to a level of activity that will help keep you at a healthy weight. Start with walking. Any activity is better than no activity at all. If you're over 35 or have any medical condition at all, check with your doctor before you start an exercise program. No matter what your age, if you haven't been exercising for some time, don't go overboard when you first start. Ease your body back into shape.

Grains and Greens

More than half of the calories in your diet should come from carbohydrates found in breads, cereals, pasta, rice, whole grains, legumes, vegetables, and fruits. One way to be sure this happens is to look at your plate whenever you sit down to eat. How much space is occupied by these foods? If it's more than half the plate, you're on the right track.

Getting Fresh

As they come from the field, grains, vegetables, and fruits are some of the most healthful foods we eat. They're naturally low in calories and fat and chock full of fiber, vitamins, and minerals. Unfortunately, some processing techniques destroy a lot of what's good about food. When grains are refined to make flour, pasta, and cereal, they often lose most of their fiber.

No Weigh!
Don't rely too much on processed and convenience foods or you'll miss out on important nutrients that only fresh foods can supply. The closer a food is to its original state, the more nutritious it tends to be because vitamins, minerals, and fiber are often lost or destroyed when food is processed.

When fruits and vegetables are canned, they lose many of their vitamins and often gain a lot of sugar and salt in the process. Frozen fruits and vegetables, on the other hand, can be just as nutritious as fresh. Try to strike a balance by including at least as many fresh foods in your diet as bottled, canned, and frozen.

Getting What You Can

It's not as hard as you think to get the five fruits and vegetables a day recommended by health experts.

➤ If you have a refrigerator at work, bring a selection of fresh fruits and vegetables for the week.

➤ Keep individual-serving size packages of raisins and dried fruit in the glove compartment of your car and in your desk drawer at work.

➤ At home, snack on fresh vegetables such as baby carrots and radishes.

➤ Take advantage of salad bars in supermarkets and delis. You can buy your vegetables raw or cooked and already cut into bite-size pieces.

➤ Add extra fresh or frozen vegetables to soups, stews, casseroles, and skillet suppers. For example, add chopped spinach to lentil soup or peas to a tuna casserole.

Cut the Fat!

Foods that are high in fat are a lot like foods that are high in sugar. They provide loads of calories but not much in the way of nutrients. Fat contains more than twice as many calories as carbohydrate or protein. If you cut back on fat, you can also cut back significantly on calories. Here are some ways you can reduce the amount of fat in your food:

➤ Use vegetable oil cooking sprays whenever you can instead of fats and oils. For instance, you don't need more than a spritz of cooking spray to sauté most foods in a nonstick skillet.

➤ Measure the fats and oils you use for cooking, rather than pour it freely.

➤ Use low-fat cooking techniques, such as steaming vegetables and poaching fish.

➤ Use herbs, spices, citrus juices, and low-fat salad dressings to flavor meats, poultry, vegetables, and grains.

➤ Try reduced-fat and fat-free versions of high-fat products you use often, such as mayonnaise, sour cream, salad dressings, and margarine spreads. Try different brands. One brand of fat-free sour cream, for instance, can taste a whole lot better than another brand.

Look Out for Saturated Fats

The Dietary Guidelines recommend a diet that's not only low in total fat but also low in saturated fat. That's the kind of fat that raises blood cholesterol more than any other kind. Meat and dairy products are the culprits when it comes to saturated fats, but that doesn't mean you shouldn't eat them. It means you should shop for the leanest cuts of meat, take the skin off your poultry before you eat it, consider reduced-fat varieties of cold cuts, hot dogs, sausages, and bacon, and use low-fat milk, yogurt, and other dairy products whenever you can.

> **No Weigh!**
> Watch out for bakery products such as cakes, cookies, doughnuts, and some muffins. They can contribute a great deal of *hidden* fat, especially saturated fat, to your diet. It's called hidden fat because you can't actually see it and it's also disguised by all the sugar that's baked in along with it.

What About Cholesterol?

This is a good place to say a word or two about cholesterol. Although most people can keep their blood cholesterol levels down by limiting the amount of total and saturated fat in their diets and by exercising, some people do have to watch the amount of cholesterol in their diets. Cholesterol is found only in animal foods such as high-fat dairy products, meat, poultry, some shellfish, and egg yolks. These are many of the same foods that are high in total fat and saturated fats. Keep in mind, however, that these are also foods that provide us with many important nutrients, so you don't want to eliminate them from your diet unless you replace them with foods that supply protein, B vitamins, calcium, and other minerals. If your blood cholesterol is affected by cholesterol in the food you eat, you have to be more careful than other people about choosing leaner meats and low-fat diary foods.

Although they tend to travel together in some of the same foods, cholesterol and fat are two completely different substances. When you take the skin off your chicken, you're taking some fat with it, but some cholesterol still remains in the meat. When fat is removed from certain foods, such as dairy products, a substantial amount of cholesterol goes with it. That's not always the case, however, so if you're watching your cholesterol, read the Nutrition Facts label found on every package of food.

Sweet Stuff

Sugar isn't quite as bad for you as some people would lead you to believe. Contrary to what you may have heard, it doesn't cause diabetes or hyperactivity. It's not at the root of your yeast infection, and you can't blame it for your weight problem. However, eating *too much* sugar doesn't help any of these conditions and beyond a certain point, it can certainly aggravate them.

Be a Sugar Sleuth

Sugar by any other name is still sugar and it sneaks into your diet in many different forms. (Those of us with a big sweet tooth don't necessarily call that a problem!) If you're concerned about the overall amount of sugar in your diet, be sure to read food labels carefully. Remember that honey, maple syrup, and molasses are all sugars and they're no more nutritious than plain, white table sugar. Be aware that if you see any of the following words on an ingredient list, you're just getting sugar that goes by another name:

➤ Corn sweetener

➤ Corn syrup or high-fructose corn syrup

➤ Fructose

➤ Dextrose

➤ Sucrose

➤ Invert sugar

➤ Malt sugar or maltose

➤ Raw sugar

➤ Turbinado sugar

➤ Fruit juice concentrate

A Rotten Sweet Tooth

NutriTip
Satisfy your sweet tooth by going to a store that sells candies by weight and buying one or two individual pieces. That's all! If you want more, you have to go all the way back to the store.

The eating patterns that help get you into trouble with your weight could also be hurting your teeth. Here's why: Bacteria in your mouth produce enamel-destroying acid for up to 30 minutes after each contact with sugar. If you sit down, eat a meal, and have dessert without brushing your teeth right away, your teeth are exposed to acid for only those 30 minutes. If you frequently snack on sweets, however, your teeth are attacked by a new wave of acid for 30 minutes every time you put a sweet food in your mouth. That can add up to many hours of acid attacks on your teeth! That's all the more reason to sit down to a satisfying meal rather than pick and snack throughout the day.

Salt Solutions

For most of the nutrients we need to be healthy, there are recommended minimum amounts we should get every day. For sodium, however, the recommendation is actually a limit. That's because most of us get a whole lot more sodium in our diets than we need, so if anything, we need to know where to stop. It's estimated that the average adult consumes between 4,000 and 6,000 mg, and most of that is from processed foods. We also get sodium from table salt.

We need a minimum of about 500 mg of sodium each day, but the recommended range for healthy people is up to 2,000 to 4,000 mg. For an idea of how much that actually is, a level teaspoon of table salt contains a little more than 2,000 mg of sodium. Even if you don't add much salt to the food you eat, you probably get more than a teaspoon's worth in the foods you eat. Most foods that are normally high in salt come in lower-salt versions.

If you're watching your salt, check food labels and compare different brands of the same type of food for sodium content. Some foods that are especially high in sodium include:

Pickles	Canned soups
Cold cuts	Potato chips
Ham	Bouillon cubes
Frankfurters	Ready-to-eat cereals
Smoked fish	Seasoned salts
Processed cheese foods	Soy sauce
Prepared frozen dinners	Worcestershire sauce

A high-sodium diet won't cause high blood pressure, but it can raise blood pressure in some people who already have the condition. If salt raises your blood pressure, you're considered "salt sensitive," but it's hard to tell who's salt sensitive and who isn't. If you do have high blood pressure, cutting down on sodium is a first-line defense. Some experts feel that everybody should have low sodium diets, regardless of blood pressure.

No Weigh!
You're not born with a particular taste for salt; you learn it along the way and you can unlearn it. The good thing about a salt habit is that it's easier to kick than other eating habits. Just don't try to go cold turkey. Cut back gradually.

If you think you need to cut back on sodium, cut back gradually rather than shock yourself into what will seem at first like a bland diet. Here are some ways you can do it:

➤ Measure the amount of salt you add in cooking and at the table and use smaller amounts.

➤ Cut the amount of salt you use in recipes by at least a third.

➤ Read the Nutrition Facts labels on the foods you buy, especially processed and canned foods, and compare the information on different brands of similar foods.

➤ Try to buy canned foods that are labeled "no salt added."

➤ Use only half the seasoning packet that comes in convenience side dishes, such as rice and noodle mixtures.

➤ Remember that fresh meat, fish, poultry, and vegetables are lower in sodium than the canned and processed varieties.

➤ Look for lower sodium varieties of bouillon, seasonings, and sauces.

167

Go Ahead, Have a Drink!

The recommendation is one drink a day for women and no more than two for men. (Men get two because they're bigger, and size matters when it comes to how much alcohol your body can handle.) That's called drinking in moderation, which is recommended if you want to stay healthy. Here's what counts as one drink:

➤ 12 ounces of beer

➤ 5 ounces of wine

➤ 1.5 ounces of 80-proof distilled spirits

NutriTip
If you drink alcohol, dilute the effect and the calories that drinks contribute to your diet by:

➤ Having your drink in a tall glass, diluted with extra juice, seltzer, or water

➤ Alternating alcoholic drinks with water or seltzer

I was once asked to give advice to a tremendously overweight woman who had a special relationship with vodka. She said she would do anything I told her to do as long as I figured 12 ounces of vodka into her daily meal plan. She actually held up an empty 12-ounce glass and said "I want this much vodka in my diet every day." I did a quick mental calculation and realized I'd have to put her on a meal plan where she would get more than 50 percent of her calories from alcohol. I didn't take the job.

You probably don't need anyone to tell you what's wrong with drinking to excess, but here's a reminder: Too much alcohol can raise your risk for high blood pressure, stroke, heart disease, certain types of cancer, accidents, and death. You could end up with cirrhosis of the liver and brain damage, not to mention malnutrition. If you're a heavy drinker, alcohol may be substituting for food you would otherwise eat, and you might not get enough nutrients in your diet. If that doesn't deter you, maybe this will: Alcohol is loaded with calories. Mixers dilute the alcohol and that's a good thing, but they can also double the calorie count. Table 14.2 gives you the score for some popular drinks.

Table 14.2 Calories in Popular Alcoholic Beverages

Alcoholic Beverage (Standard Serving Size)	Approximate Calories
Beer (12 oz.)	150
Light beer (12 oz.)	100
Champagne (5 oz.)	133
Wine, red or white (5 oz.)	105
Vodka/Gin/Rum/Whiskey (1.5 oz.)	100–125
Daiquiri (4.5 oz.)	250
Martini (2.5 oz.)	155
Pina colada (4.5 oz.)	260

Alcoholic Beverage (Standard Serving Size)	Approximate Calories
Screwdriver (7 oz.)	175
Tequila sunrise (5.5 oz.)	190

The Least You Need to Know

➤ The best way to keep your diet interesting and get all the nutrients you need is to eat a wide variety of foods.

➤ The way to maintain a healthy weight is to balance the amount of calories you consume from food and drinks with enough exercise every day.

➤ More than half the calories in a healthy diet should come from carbohydrates found in grains, vegetables, and fruit.

➤ Because fat contains more than twice as many calories as carbohydrate and protein, cutting back on fat can help you cut back on the amount of calories you get in your diet.

➤ Although sugar isn't as bad as some people make it out to be, too much of the sweet stuff can make you feel sick and contribute to your weight problem.

➤ You probably get more than enough salt in your diet even if you don't add any at the table.

➤ A drink or two might not harm your health, but keep in mind that alcoholic beverages can add a significant number of unnecessary calories to your diet.

Part 5
Exercise 101

If you think exercise is hard work, you're right. So's life! But life is easier when you're mentally and physically fit. Nothing does more to get your mind and body into shape than a daily dose of exercise.

Even hard work can be fun if you like what you do, so these next few chapters are filled with ideas for fun ways to exercise. Think of this part as your "warm-up" to a workout that will leave you feeling stronger, leaner, and more energized. By the end of this part, you'll have enough information and motivation to plan an exercise program you can look forward to following.

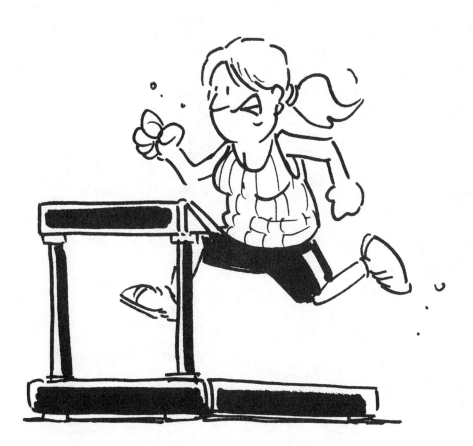

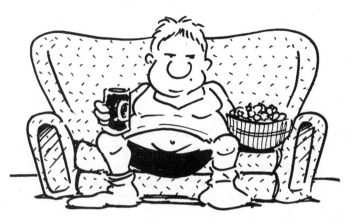

Chapter 15

Why Exercise?

In This Chapter

➤ Exercising to stay fit

➤ The health benefits of working out

➤ Getting lean

➤ Fitting exercise into your schedule

Some people can't even *say* the word *exercise* without making a funny face. "Can't I just eat less?," they beg. Sure, you can lose pounds by eating less food. *If* you can eat less food, that is. Even if you *could* stay on a low-calorie diet forever, I don't advise it. When you lose weight only by dieting, you lose muscle, too, and that's not the healthiest way to lose weight. You want to hold on to your muscle and you do that by exercising.

To be honest, it came as a surprise when I first learned that exercise is as important as food when it comes to losing weight and staying fit. As a nutritionist, I used to think food was the answer to everything. Wrong! It's only the answer to half of everything! The key to weight control is balancing the amount of food you eat with enough activity to burn off any extra calories before they settle in as body fat. The more extra calories, the more exercise you need.

This chapter gives you a lot of good reasons to start moving toward a fit and healthy future—right now!

The ABCs of Fitness

When you're fit, you look and feel the best you can. You're mentally alert and physically capable of performing work. You have energy to spare so you're able to enjoy activities outside of work. You're healthy.

Of course, everyone's appropriate level of fitness is different due to age, sex, heredity, and personal eating and exercise habits. When you want to improve your fitness level, your focus must be on maintaining a healthy weight because that's where you have the power to change things. For most people, exercise plays a huge role in weight control. *People who successfully maintain a healthy weight after losing weight or who never really have a problem with weight tend to be people who exercise often.*

No Weigh!
You don't always lose weight when you start to exercise. Because you're building muscle and muscle weighs more than fat, you might actually gain a pound or two. Never fear! You'll lose inches even if you don't lose pounds and your shape will change. You'll start fitting into smaller clothes. You'll look better and you'll be healthier.

Exercise helps control your weight because it uses extra calories that otherwise get stored in your body as fat. Obviously, the amount of exercise you need to control your weight depends on how much you eat. It also depends on the type of exercise you choose to do. Any physical work you do—such as running, gardening, lifting boxes, or dancing—uses calories. The more active you are, the more calories you'll use. But exercise does more for your overall fitness level than burn calories. Exercise can also:

➤ Build muscle

➤ Boost energy

➤ Improve your mood

➤ Suppress your appetite

➤ Reduce the effects of stress

➤ Improve your posture

➤ Encourage other positive lifestyle changes

➤ Condition your heart

➤ Strengthen your bones

➤ Lengthen your life

Off to a Good Start

If exercise is a brand new thing for you, start slow and add just a few minutes more activity every day. A ten-minute walk is a lot better than no walk at all—or a ten-minute swim. Next week, walk or swim for 12 minutes. You want to start getting into a regular exercise routine, so choose an exercise you're comfortable with, and do it at a time that suits your schedule. Gradually, over time, increase the length and pace of your workout.

Your ultimate goal is to get at least 30 minutes of steady, moderate exercise at least 5 times a week. There may be reasons why you can't reach that goal, however. Second best: Get your 30 minutes of exercise a day, 5 or 10 minutes at a time, or aim for 30 minutes 3 to 4 times a week.

Advice from Losers

"I started running again after putting on 30 pounds. But I was so out of shape I had to run 1 minute, then walk 9 minutes. I repeated that cycle for 40 minutes. The next week I ran 2 minutes, walked 8 and repeated that for 40 minutes. The hard part was when I got to 5 minutes and 5 minutes. I was really tempted to blow the program and try to run the whole time. But I knew it was too soon and I could hurt myself or exhaust myself and give up. I kept increasing my running time each week until I was running the full 40 minutes again. I lost the weight, and I'm still running!"

—Christopher C.

Choose activities you truly enjoy. If you like to be part of a group, try to join a local soccer, softball, or basketball team. Take classes at the gym. If exercise is your time to be alone, walking, running, riding a bike, or swimming might be your choice. Exercise is serious stuff, but that doesn't mean it can't be fun. Play games! Volleyball, Frisbee, golf, tennis, and even croquet all count as exercise. Take a hike, climb a mountain, or walk new trails, even if your "trails" are simply suburban back roads. Exploring new territory will help keep walking and other light exercise interesting.

Unless you spend most of every day cleaning or repairing your home, you won't burn a significant number of calories doing housework, but everyday activities still count as exercise. Mopping floors, scraping paint, and cleaning out cabinets all involve stretching and bending. You might even work up a light sweat. Take advantage of any opportunity to move. So what if you drive to the mall and the parking lot is practically full? Walk the distance and you've done ten extra minutes of exercise. Once you're fit, you'll feel less tired overall, and you'll actually enjoy any opportunity you get to add an extra mini-workout to your day.

Guru's Corner

"People who don't exercise always ask me, 'What's the best exercise to do to lose weight?' Almost all activity burns energy, and usually the issue is not *what* exercise is being done but *if* exercise is being done. So my answer to which exercise is best for weight loss is, 'The one that you will do.'"

—Darrell Vogel, Psy.D., Behavioral Director, Obesity Consultation Center, New England Medical Center, Boston, Massachusetts

If you're over 40 or have any health conditions, you should check with your doctor before you start a moderate or intense exercise program. Be sure your doctor is aware if you have any of the following problems:

Chest pains

Heart or lung disease

Dizzy or fainting spells

Diabetes

High blood pressure

Breathlessness or wheezing after mild exertion

Arthritis

Back or leg pain

Finding Motivation

If you need other people to keep you motivated, find a gym buddy to work out with or a running partner to jog with or find a group activity such as a sport or an aerobics class. If you join a gym, be sure it's convenient to where you live or work so it's easy to get there. Here are some sure ways to stay motivated:

➤ Pick a time of day that works best for you. Some people prefer to get their exercise over with first thing in the morning. Others prefer to exercise in the afternoon and use their workout to help relieve the stress of the day. Some people choose to exercise during those high-risk times when they are usually prone to overeating or snacking.

➤ Don't let exercise get boring. Vary your workout routine to keep it interesting.

➤ Challenge yourself. Just keep thinking how good you'll feel *afterward*.

➤ Think about the improvements you're making to your physical and mental health.

➤ Use the reward system. Whenever you add more time to your exercise routine or increase the pace, consider it a milestone and reward yourself with a gift. It can be a theater ticket, a new CD, or anything else that isn't food.

Weather Watch

If you exercise outdoors, weather can get in the way of a successful workout. When the humidity is high, sweat doesn't evaporate from your body as easily as in dry weather.

Wear lightweight fabrics when you exercise in hot weather to allow sweat to evaporate. Wear white and light-colored clothes to reflect the heat. You might want to wear a lightweight baseball cap or visor to keep the sun off your head and out of your face. Drink a cup of water 20 or 30 minutes before exercising in hot weather, about $1/2$ cup of water every 10 or 15 minutes while you exercise, and another cup or more during the 30 minutes following exercise.

It's just as important to drink enough fluids in cold weather as it is in hot weather. You lose more water vapor when you exhale and you excrete more fluids in cold weather. Wear layers of clothing so you can remove them as your body temperature increases during exercise and replace them when you stop to rest. Wear a hat when you exercise outdoors and particularly when you stop to rest so you don't lose heat through your head.

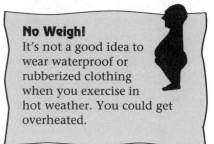

No Weigh!
It's not a good idea to wear waterproof or rubberized clothing when you exercise in hot weather. You could get overheated.

Exercise in Good Health

Many people suffer from overweight and illnesses that could be improved or prevented by regular exercise. Exercise can also improve your chances of living longer. If you work out most days of the week, you'll be better able to control your weight, and you'll also reduce your risk of developing chronic disease such as:

Heart disease   Diabetes

High blood pressure   Osteoporosis

Exercise Styles

There are two types of exercise: aerobic and nonaerobic. We'll get into them in more detail in Chapter 17, "Move It!" but for now you should at least know the difference between the two and what each can do for you.

➤ Aerobic means "with oxygen." During aerobic exercise such as running or biking, oxygen is taken into your body and delivered to your body cells. How effectively that happens is a measure of your aerobic fitness.

➤ Anaerobic or nonaerobic means without oxygen. Anaerobic exercise is any activity that's not steady or not fast enough to be aerobic, such as bowling or slow dancing.

Aerobic exercise is important for overall health and fitness and it helps burns calories while you're exercising. However, the trend in exercising for weight control is moving toward strength training with weights and resistance. Strength training builds muscle and the more muscle you build, the better able you are to burn fat. That's because muscle is more "metabolically active" in your body than fat. That means muscle cells burn calories and produce energy, and they continue to burn calories well after you stop exercising.

If you exercise aerobically for at least 20 or 30 minutes, three times a week, you'll strengthen your heart. Regular exercise can also lower the cholesterol in your blood and reduce your blood pressure if you already have high blood pressure. That reduces your risk of heart disease and stroke. Weight-bearing exercise helps build and maintain healthy bones, muscles, and joints. This is especially important for older men and women who want to stay strong and steady and reduce their risk of developing osteoporosis.

Healthy Body, Healthy Mind

The psychological benefits of exercise motivate a lot of people to get up off their butts and move. Many people use exercise as a stress-buster and mood elevator. Besides the boost in self-esteem and body image that goes hand-in-hand with being fit, exercise can help you feel less anxious or depressed. One study found that people who normally exercise 6 or 7 times a week for at least 45 minutes felt less vigorous and more anxious, tense, and depressed after just one day of skipping their exercise routines. When they started working out again, they immediately felt better.

If stress is at the core of your overeating, you might get multiple benefits from adding mind-body exercises such as yoga and t'ai chi to the workout routine you develop. There are studios that specialize in yoga and t'ai chi classes and many health clubs now offer classes in both. Although these are two completely different types of exercises, both are meditative in nature and they have a common goal of improving both physical and mental well-being:

➤ Yoga originated in India but is now practiced all over the world. Yoga exercises can help you develop physical strength, endurance, and flexibility. At the same time, the focus in a yoga class is on self-awareness and mental well-being. Yoga combines physical poses with breathing and relaxation techniques. The goal is a quiet mind in a physically healthy body.

➤ T'ai chi is a form of Chinese martial arts that is used to reduce stress. Although it began as a self-defense system, the t'ai chi methods practiced in the West are more often like a moving form of yoga. T'ai chi consists of very slow, graceful, and precise movements that teach balance and alignment. The exercises can help improve your posture, lower body strength, and coordination at the same time they teach you to relax your mind.

The Meaning of Lean

You've heard the term lean body mass? Here's what it means: Take your weight and subtract your fat, and what's left is your lean body mass. That includes muscle, bones, and organs. Here's why it's important: The more lean mass you have, the higher your metabolic rate and the better you burn calories. The more muscle power you have, the stronger you are and the easier it is to be more active.

It's important to exercise different parts of your body in different ways so that you reach all the different muscle groups. The illustration on the following page shows you where your different muscles are located on your body and what they look like.

When you're trying to lose weight, you exercise to hold on to your muscle while you lose fat. If all you do to lose weight is cut back on the amount of food you eat, you'll lose healthy muscle tissue along with fat. When you lose muscle, you lose some of your ability to burn calories efficiently.

Basically, you exercise to improve your

> **Guru's Corner**
> "A pear-shaped person who starts to eat better and exercise but only does aerobics simply becomes a smaller pear. Weight training is an important part of any exercise program because it not only helps you maintain a higher metabolism, it can actually help modify your body shape. Aerobics strengthen your heart but weight training helps tone up problem areas for a more balanced shape."
>
> —Angela Redden, M.S., Exercise Physiologist, Memphis, Tennessee

➤ Endurance. Cardiorespiratory endurance allows oxygen and nutrients to be delivered to your body cells for longer periods of time. Long runs are one way to build up cardiovascular endurance. You also want to build up muscular endurance. Push-ups are a good example of an exercise that builds muscular endurance.

➤ Strength. Your strength is measured by the amount of force your muscles can exert in a single effort. Different weight-lifting and weight-bearing exercises strengthen your different muscle groups.

➤ Flexibility. To move your joints and use your muscles through their full range of motion, you need good flexibility. The more flexible you are, the less chance you have of hurting yourself. Good flexibility also leads to better posture and better exercise performance. Yoga, t'ai chi, and stretching routines all help improve flexibility and reduce muscle tension. When you do stretching exercises, it's important not to bounce. Instead, hold the stretch for 10 to 15 seconds.

*Your muscular
system*

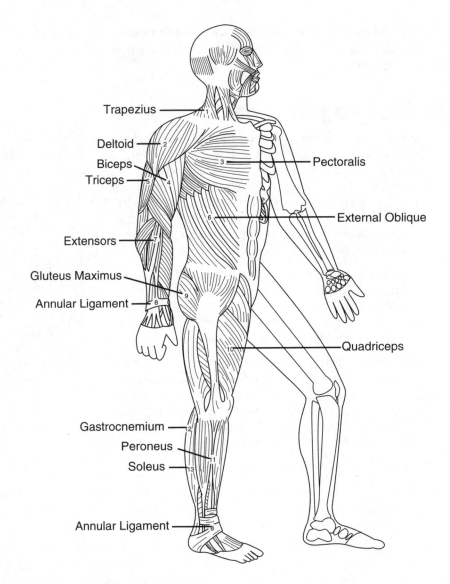

Trapezius

Deltoid

Biceps

Triceps

Pectoralis

External Oblique

Extensors

Gluteus Maximus

Annular Ligament

Quadriceps

Gastrocnemium

Peroneus

Soleus

Annular Ligament

Your Workout Schedule

Pick a specific time of day that's best for you to exercise and try to stick with it. That way, you'll develop a routine and exercise can more easily become a regular habit. You can start exercising just a few days a week and then, little-by-little, start setting higher goals. Ideally, your total weekly exercise program will include workouts for endurance, strength, and flexibility, but be realistic. Do what you can, and don't set yourself up for failure by setting goals you can't reach. That means ultimately finding time in your workout schedule for

➤ Five to ten minutes of warm-up exercises such as walking, easy jogging, and arm and leg rotations before *every* workout. Warm-up exercises reduce the risk of injury. They actually increase the temperature in your muscles and connective tissue and send blood to the area with the extra oxygen needed for exercise. Your warm-up can include body motions similar to those you'll be using in your actual exercise, such as a slow swim before swimming or slow biking before biking.

➤ Twenty to thirty minutes of ongoing aerobic activity at least three times a week.

➤ Twenty minutes of lifting weights, at least twice a week, to exercise your major muscle groups.

➤ Thirty minutes of calisthenics, sit-ups, push-ups, pull-ups, and weight-bearing exercises at least three times a week to build muscular endurance.

➤ Ten minutes of slow stretching every day, following warm-up or combined with cooling down exercises.

➤ Five to ten minutes of cool-down exercise such as walking.

> **No Weigh!**
> Don't overexercise with weights. You have to rest and let your muscles recover at least a day after doing resistance exercises. Every other day, alternate aerobic and strengthening exercises, such as running and weight lifting.

The Least You Need to Know

➤ Exercise plays a big role in weight and fat control, which help determine your fitness level.

➤ If you haven't been exercising up until now, start slow. Even a few minutes a day is a big improvement if you haven't been doing any exercise at all.

➤ In addition to helping you control your weight, exercise can help reduce your risk of developing heart disease, diabetes, high blood pressure, and osteoporosis.

➤ Different types of exercise provide different health benefits. That's why it's beneficial to incorporate both aerobic and strengthening exercises into your fitness plan.

➤ If you're over 40 or have any medical problems, check with your doctor before you begin any new exercise program.

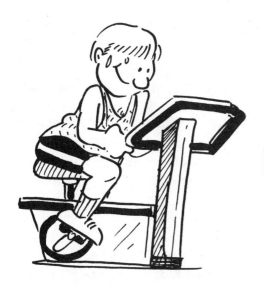

Chapter 16

Exercise Options

In This Chapter

➤ What to think about before you join a health club or gym

➤ Why not take up a sport?

➤ Dancing for fitness

➤ Workout options for home bodies

Feel like sliding, spinning, or hip-hopping tonight? You can step out to a nightclub, but if that's not your thing, head for a health club! This chapter tells you what to look for when you're choosing a gym and what to expect when you get there. Gone are the days when exercise meant boring, repetitive squats and lifts. Exercise classes are as tough as they ever were, but now they're a lot more fun and sometimes, you hardly know you're working.

If the gym's not your thing either, you might be the sporting type. This chapter gives you a lot of different exercise options, including tips for getting a great workout at home.

How to Join a Gym

One of the most important first considerations you have when joining a gym or health club is convenience. Is it close to your home or your job so that you can get there easily enough? If not, the club's location can become an excuse for not exercising. If it's close to work, will be you able to work out during your lunch hour? If not, you could just as easily pick a gym close to home because you'll be exercising before or after work and possibly on weekends. You might want to join a gym where you have friends who are members so you can work out together and keep each other motivated. Here are some other things to consider before you lay your money down:

➤ Cost. Can you afford to join this gym? Will you use the services you're paying for? If your membership fee helps support spa services such as saunas, steam rooms, and tanning salons or a climbing wall that you'll never use, it might make more sense to join a less expensive gym. Also be sure you're ready to commit to a long-term plan before you sign up for one.

➤ Comfort. Some gyms seem to attract serious body-building or *Baywatch* types, and that can be intimidating to a mere mortal. Be sure you feel comfortable in the gym's environment.

➤ Class schedule. Does this gym offer classes you want to take that are at your fitness level and at times that are convenient for you?

➤ Variety. Does this gym offer a wide variety of the types of classes or equipment you're interested in? For example, if you want to learn how to work out with free weights, are there different types of body sculpting classes at times that are convenient for you? If you're looking for aerobic workouts, are there a variety of step, spinning, and dance classes?

➤ Services. Does the gym offer fitness testing? Are personal trainers available? Can you rent a locker?

➤ Trainer certification. Are the trainers certified by a nationally recognized organization? Such organizations include the American Council on Exercise (ACE), the Aerobics and Fitness Association of America (AFAA), and the American College of Sports Medicine (ACSM).

➤ Baby-sitting. Does this gym offer baby-sitting services if you need them? If so, are you completely comfortable with the qualifications of the caregivers and the playroom itself?

Advice from Losers

"Six years ago I was 45 pounds overweight and when I finally decided to do something about it, I hired a personal trainer at my gym. I continued to eat whenever I was hungry, but I started eating more low-fat foods. I met with my trainer twice a week to learn how to strength-train correctly. I started taking aerobics classes at the same time, and eventually worked my way up to five or six days of aerobics and four days of strength training. I liked my trainer and my workout so much that I left the pharmaceutical sales field to become a certified trainer myself!"

—Sue K.

Step, Slide, Spin, or Sculpt

Deciding which classes to take at the gym is a matter of personal choice. It depends on the type of movements you enjoy and what your exercise goal is, as well as your fitness level. You might have to try a few classes before you settle on the type of exercise that suits your needs and your personality. When you belong to a large health club that offers many class choices, you might base your decision on the personality and skill level of the instructor. Exercise classes go in and out of style as more and more programs are developed to keep workouts from getting boring. As new fitness products are developed, new classes are designed around them. Here are some brief descriptions of routine classes offered at many health clubs:

➤ Body sculpting involves movements that condition your muscles with resistance training and hand weights.

➤ Abs classes concentrate on strengthening and shaping the abdominal area, and they are often shorter in length than other classes. Sometimes "abs" are combined with butt and thigh exercises in a full-length class.

➤ Step is a low-impact, high-intensity workout that involves stepping up and down on an adjustable-level platform.

➤ Box aerobics is an aerobics class that incorporates boxing moves.

➤ Cardio-step is a high-intensity step class that includes other aerobic exercises.

➤ Slide is an aerobic workout that involves sliding from side-to-side on a specially designed mat, wearing special shoe coverings. Slide is usually combined with step or other strength-training techniques.

➤ High-low impact aerobics combines high-impact movements with low-impact movements.

➤ Funk aerobics is an aerobic dance class.

➤ Spinning is a high-intensity, no-impact aerobic workout on specially designed stationary bikes.

NutriTip
Bring a water bottle to every class. You need to drink water before, during, and after every workout, especially if it's an aerobic workout.

Fitness Instructors

When you first join a gym, it pays to check out different classes and different teachers to see which ones are best for you. The American Council on Exercise suggests that when you choose a class, look for an instructor who is certified by a nationally

No Weigh!
Don't be afraid to talk to an exercise instructor. Let him or her know that you're new to the gym or new to the class. A good instructor will ease you into the class routine and help you feel more comfortable about trying something new and getting the most out of your workout.

recognized certifying organization. That way, you're more assured of a safe, effective workout. A good instructor will make you feel welcome by learning your name and making eye contact with you throughout the session. You should feel like you're in a safe, noncompetitive environment where the focus is on good health, not just good looks. Stick with instructors who give thorough demonstrations and explain the benefits of each exercise.

Gym Etiquette

There's an acceptable way to behave in gyms in the same way that there's an acceptable way to behave at work, school, and everywhere else. Here are a few of the unwritten rules that gym visitors are expected to follow:

➤ Use a towel to wipe off exercise equipment after you've used it so that no one else has to sit in your sweat.

➤ Don't hog the equipment, especially during busy times at the gym. Allow other exercisers to work in between your sets. Often there are sign-up sheets for popular machines. If you're late, you lose. Use the machine only for your allotted time period.

➤ Most exercisers want to be able to hear the instructor and focus on their workout, so don't make any unnecessary noise.

➤ Latecomers to a class are very distracting to other exercisers. If you can't slip quietly into the back row, wait for another class.

➤ When you're finished with weights and equipment, put them back where you found them.

➤ Don't spread your personal clutter around for others to clean up or trip over.

If you live in an area where there aren't many gyms to choose from, be sure the gym you're considering is up to par. If you have any doubts, or if you're just not a "joiner," find another way to exercise, such as road running, bicycling, or working out in your own home. You don't need a gym membership to get fit.

What a Sport!

Playing sports usually means investing in special equipment or at the very least, special attire. If you like teamwork and competition, a group sport such as softball or volleyball might be the workout choice for you. Regular aerobic, strength-training, and stretching exercises can help keep you in shape for sports if they strengthen the muscles you use for the sport and increase your flexibility.

On the Green

You'll walk a good 3 to 4 miles in the course of an 18-hole golf game, so you need good endurance. You also need good flexibility in your shoulders, legs, and midsection. It helps to have good upper-body strength to hit the ball as far as it has to go. Stretching and strength-training exercises can help you get in shape for your game, and of course, you'll become more conditioned as you play. Take lessons, or go to a golf camp, and then practice, practice, practice! To be a good golfer, you'll need:

➤ Golf clubs

➤ Golf club bag

➤ Golf glove

➤ Golf balls

➤ Golf tees

➤ Golf shoes

> **Guru's Corner**
>
> "When exercise and sports are part of your plan to lose weight, eat most of your food during the day and be reasonable at night. That way, you'll have lots of energy for your workout, you'll burn off the calories when you exercise, and you'll already have had enough food so you won't be so tempted to overeat at night."
>
> —Nancy Clark, M.S., R.D., nutritionist at SportsMedicine, Brookline, MA, and author of *Nancy Clark's Sports Nutrition Guidebook*, Second ed. (Human Kinetics, 1997)

Tennis, Anyone?

Tennis is an aerobic sport that gives your butt and calves a particularly good workout once you learn how to play. When tennis is played by two people, it's called "singles," and when it's played by four people, it's called "doubles." You get a better workout when you play singles because you're moving more often. It pays to take basic lessons from a tennis pro. In addition to lessons, you'll need:

➤ Tennis shoes

➤ A tennis racket

➤ Tennis balls

Take a Dive!

Swimming is an aerobic exercise that can also give you a good upper-body workout. If you don't already know how to swim, take lessons. When you know the correct way to swim, it's more fun and a more effective exercise. Besides basic swimming, there are many water sports you can play to keep a wet workout interesting. For example, water jogging is a non-impact way to get a run. A specially designed vest keeps you upright and afloat while you "jog." Just walking in the shallow end of a pool is a great exercise. For basic swimming, you'll need:

➤ A bathing suit (one-piece tank for women)

➤ A swim cap

➤ Goggles (optional)

In-line Skating

No Weigh!
Don't judge your workout by the amount of sweat you produce. Sweat is your body's way of cooling off when you start to overheat, but it's not necessarily an indicator of how hard you're working.

Once you can skate at a moderately speedy pace, you'll get a decent aerobic workout from skating. Like ice skating, in-line skating is also great for toning up your butt, hips, and thighs. Before you get into any of the fancy moves you see the pros doing on TV, however, practice skating in an empty lot or anywhere you can find a lot of flat wide-open space. Protective gear is essential for this sport. Besides skates, you'll need:

➤ Wrist and elbow guards

➤ Knee pads

➤ A helmet

Down the Slopes

You have to get into shape to ski and know what you're doing, or you can really hurt yourself—or others. A friend of mine suffered more than a little embarrassment when, after landing on her butt more than half a dozen times, she was asked by the ski patrol to remove her skis and walk down the side of an intermediate-level hill she had no business tackling to begin with.

Don't let that happen to you. To ski, you need to develop your balance and coordination, as well as your strength and endurance. According to the experts at the American Council on Exercise, bouncing two tennis balls at once will improve your coordination. They also recommend squats and lunges for building lower-body strength and abdominal crunches to create a solid "core" for balance and agility. If you're unfamiliar with a particular ski resort, call and ask about the difficulty of their runs before you go. Wherever you go to ski, you can usually rent equipment. To ski, you need:

➤ Skis

➤ Poles

➤ Boots

➤ Ski clothing

Off the Charts

Exercise is first and foremost about getting fit and healthy. It's also about burning calories and losing weight. All sports and other physical activities help improve your fitness level, but some burn up a lot more calories than others. Remember: The more you weigh, the more calories you burn performing any exercise because the extra weight forces you to work harder. Table 16.1 shows how some popular sports and activities compare when it comes to burning calories. Find your favorite and then move your finger across to the weight closest to yours to see how many calories you'll burn per minute at that activity.

NutriTip
You'll burn more calories if you exercise at a moderate pace for a longer period of time than if you exercise at an overly intense pace for a shorter period of time.

Table 16.1 Calories Used per Minute

Activity	120 lbs.	140 lbs.	160 lbs.	180 lbs.
Basketball	7.5	8.8	10.0	11.3
Bowling	1.2	1.4	1.6	1.9
Cycling (10 mph)	5.5	6.4	7.3	8.2
Dancing (aerobic)	7.4	8.6	9.8	11.1
Dancing (social)	2.9	3.3	3.7	4.2
Gardening	5.0	5.9	6.7	7.5
Golf, carry clubs	4.6	5.4	6.2	7.0
Golf, power cart	2.1	2.5	2.8	3.2
Hiking	4.5	5.2	6.0	6.7
In-line skating	5.9	6.9	7.9	8.8
Jogging	9.3	10.8	12.4	13.9
Running	11.4	13.2	15.1	17.0
Sitting quietly	1.2	1.3	1.5	1.7
Skiing, cross-country	7.5	8.8	10.0	11.3
Skiing, water or downhill	5.7	6.6	7.6	8.5
Swimming, moderate	7.8	9.0	10.3	11.6
Tennis	6.0	6.9	7.9	8.9
Walking	6.5	7.6	8.7	9.7
Weight training	6.6	7.6	8.7	9.8

Reprinted with permission from the American Council on Exercise from ACE Fit Facts.

Dance Your Way to Fitness

Just as I turned off the TV to start working on this chapter, I heard a news flash announcing that disco dancing is coming back. Another time I might have rolled my eyes and said "Why?" to no one in particular. Instead I thought, "Wow, that's great because it's such good exercise." Fast dancing is right up there on the A-list of aerobic activities. You can burn up more than 400 calories in an hour, and what could be more fun?

No Weigh!
Don't wear restrictive clothing for dancing, and skip the high heels unless you have a lot of experience. If you want dancing to give you a good workout, you have to be free to move.

Dancing is an exercise almost anyone can do anytime, anywhere. Think about it. There's practically no excuse *not* to dance! You can go out and dance at a studio, a gym, or a nightclub. You can dance when you're traveling, when you're with someone else, or when you're alone. You can dance when you're young and when you're old. If you're intimidated by public workouts, dancing is the perfect exercise to do at home. Put on some music and prance around your living room, acting out your fantasy of becoming a famous rock star or prima ballerina. Rent an instructional video and teach yourself some actual dance steps.

There are many different kinds of dances you can learn, from ballet to tap dancing to salsa. Here are a few other classics to consider:

Latin-American dances	Contra dancing
Samba	Line dancing
Rumba	Circle mixers
Paso doble	Standard ballroom dances
Cha cha	Viennese waltz
Jive	Modern waltz
American country dances	Tango
Square dancing	Slow fox-trot
	Quickstep

Learn how to dance and you can tango off as many calories as you would swimming, skating, or riding a bike. Of course, that's from vigorous dancing, but even slower, steadier dancing can help keep you get fit and strengthen your bones. When you're dancing, you're constantly moving and covering a great distance without even noticing because you're having so much fun at the same time. Of course, if you want to see fitness benefits from dancing, the trick, as with any exercise, is to do it often and do it regularly.

Once you learn a few basic moves, dancing is just a matter of practice. Dance groups often meet in community centers, church basements, YMCAs, and YWCAs. Many gyms offer classes, although they may be limited to aerobic and jazz or funk-style dancing. To take formal dance lessons, find the nearest dance studio in your area or check with your local parks and recreation bureau. The United States Amateur Ballroom Dancers Association (USABDA) has a network of chapters in more than 120 cities around the country. Each chapter sponsors regular social dances that are open to the public, and they work with professional instructors in the area to provide group lessons at these dances. To find a chapter in your area, contact

U.S. Amateur Ballroom Dancers Association
P.O. Box 128
New Freedom, PA 17349
(800) 447-9047

Exercising at Home

If you're not a "gym body," you can still be an exercising "home body." You can spend from $20 to $2,000 dollars to equip a home gym, depending on the type of exercise you like to do and the equipment required to do it correctly. On the low end, you might decide that all you need to work out at home is a jump rope and set of elastic resistance bands. At the other extreme, you might want to turn your entire basement into a home gym and equip it with a couple of machines and a graduated set of free weights. Besides money considerations, a lot depends on how much room you have in your home and how much discipline you have to work out on your own. Do yourself a favor and research before buying exercise equipment or expensive gear. Publications such as *Consumer Reports*, *Shape*, and other fitness magazines often feature buyers' guides that compare different brands and types of exercise items. Following is a basic menu of aerobic and strength training equipment you might want to consider:

> **NutriTip**
> The caffeine in a single cup of coffee or tea can help you stay alert while you exercise and might even enhance your workout. Just remember that caffeine is a diuretic that causes you to lose fluids that must be replaced.

For Aerobic Exercises	*For Strength Training and Toning*
Treadmill	Free weights
Stationary bike	Weight machines
Stair climber	Specific body part equipment such as ab roller
Rowing machine	Elastic bands or tubes
Cross-country machine	Body balls
Step platform (adjustable height)	
Jump rope	

Buying Equipment

The best piece of advice anyone can give you about buying major exercise equipment is do your research. Talk to people who own the equipment you're thinking about buying in addition to talking to dealers. If you know any fitness professionals, talk to them about respected brand names. Be sure you feel comfortable with the quality and design of the machine. To find equipment that's right for you, follow these guidelines from the Aerobics and Fitness Association of America (AFAA):

No Weigh!
Don't let anyone pressure you into buying expensive or inappropriate exercise equipment before you really know what you want. Go out and gather information, and then go home and sleep on it before you make a decision.

➤ Go into a store or showroom and try the equipment. Look for proper fit or feel, smooth moving parts, sturdy, stable construction, and delivery of what's offered.

➤ Check that the product comes with a long-term warranty ensuring that the manufacturer will repair or replace any faulty parts for up to a year after you buy the equipment. Even better is a money-back guarantee that lets you test the product and return it for a full refund if you're not happy with it.

➤ Compare prices. Price is often, but not always, an indicator of quality. Comparing prices helps you figure out an average range for a particular type of exercise equipment.

Exercise Video Picks

Before you invest in major machinery, you might want to start with an exercise video you can follow at home. Stick with videos that feature well-established instructors who have built a solid reputation in the exercise field. Within the same series of video titles, such as the "Steel" series (*Buns of Steel, Abs of Steel,* and so on), you may prefer some instructors over others. If you're not familiar with a video instructor or series, get recommendations from friends who've used exercise videos. Some of the most popular and reliable videos and instructors include:

The Firm series	Kathy Smith
The Crunch series	Donna Richardson
Richard Simmons	Karen Voight
	The "Steel" series

One of the largest collections of exercise videos is available at Collage Video in Minneapolis. Even if you don't know what you want, you can call them and ask a consultant for advice. Be sure to ask about the skill level required and the style of the instructor on any video the consultant recommends. Also, check to be sure the video exercises don't require additional equipment you're not prepared to buy. Collage caries videos for kids, seniors, pregnant women, and people with back problems. You can order just about any title you're looking for or simply call for a copy of their catalog at (800) 433-6769.

The Least You Need to Know

➤ If you decide to join a gym, choose one that has a convenient location and all the classes and services you require.

➤ The best exercise instructors and trainers are certified by a nationally recognized organization such as the American Council on Exercise (ACE), the Aerobics and Fitness Association of America (AFAA), or the American College of Sports Medicine (ACSM).

➤ Playing sports and dancing are fun ways to work out and give you the same benefits as any other exercise if you practice them on a regular basis.

➤ Compare different brands and styles of home-gym equipment and thoroughly test any machine you're considering before you make a make a purchase.

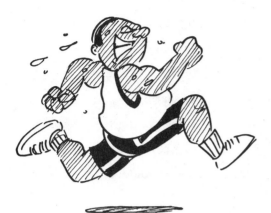

Chapter 17

Move It!

In This Chapter

➤ The ABCs of aerobic exercise

➤ Weight training for muscle strength

➤ Why cross-training is so important

➤ Walking your way to fitness

➤ Keeping track of your progress

Even though you're just one body, you've got a lot of different body parts that need working out. Some parts, such as your heart, get the most benefit from uninterrupted aerobic exercise such as what you get from dancing and running. Other parts, such as your muscles, get stronger from strength training exercises like push-ups and pumping iron.

This chapter shows you how to be as fit as you can be. Now, don't get overwhelmed! What's most important is that you get yourself started and it's perfectly okay to start off slow.

All About Aerobics

Whenever a workout gets your pulse rate up to training level and keeps it there for at least 20 minutes, you're doing an aerobic exercise. Exercises that are considered aerobic include:

Fast walking	Jogging
Running	Jumping rope
Rowing	Riding a bicycle
Cross-country skiing	Ice skating
Roller skating	Inline skating
Swimming	Stair climbing
Aerobic or disco dancing	Playing handball, racquetball, or squash

Warming Up

The best warm-up exercises use the same muscles that you'll be using when you get to the actual exercise. A warm-up starts you off slow. You can warm up for bicycling with a slow bike ride or warm up for a run with a walk and a slow jog. Warm-ups usually last five to ten minutes.

Your Training Heart Rate

The fitness benefit you get from aerobic exercise depends on how much oxygen your body uses while you work out. To get the most benefit, you have to take in more oxygen than usual and your heart has to beat faster to get that oxygen into your muscles. According to the Aerobics and Fitness Association of America (AFAA), aerobic exercise should be maintained for a minimum of 20 to 30 minutes, with your heart rate maintained at 55 to 85 percent of your estimated maximum heart rate, or the fastest your heart is able to beat.

No Weigh!
Never start your exercise sessions by stretching. Stretching a cold muscle can lead to tearing. You can stretch *after* you warm up or while you're cooling down.

The formula for figuring out your training heart rate range (THRR) is

THRR = 220 – your age × .55 to .85

For example, here's how to use the formula if you're 36 years old:

220 – 36 = 184

184 × .55 = 101

101 = 55 percent of your estimated maximum heart rate, or the low end of your training range.

$184 \times .85 = 156$

156 = 85 percent of your estimated maximum heart rate, or the high end of your training range.

At age 36, your THRR is 101 to 156 beats per minute.

The most accurate way to determine if you're within your range is with a pulse/heart monitor. If you don't have one, you can stop exercising and count the pulse beats at your wrist or neck for 15 seconds. Multiply the number of beats by four. That's your beats-per-minute. Are you within your training heart rate zone? If your heart is beating slower, you need to exercise a little harder. If your heart is beating faster than your training rate, you need to slow down.

> **No Weigh!**
> Stop exercising if you have difficulty breathing or feel faint or weak. That means you're exercising too hard and could hurt yourself. You should be able to hold a conversation while you exercise.

When you first start to exercise, your goal is to get your heart rate up to the low end of your training range. You might not even be in the range at first. That's okay. Keep exercising at a comfortable pace, and you'll get there. As you become more fit, your goal will be to get to the top of your range.

Cooling Down

You have to do cool-down exercises for the sake of your heart. Rather than stop suddenly and have your heart rate drop quickly, continue with the same workout but at a slower stride. This allows your heartbeat to slowly drop back to its normal rate.

Cooling down is like warming up in reverse. If you've been running or jogging, bring it down to a slow jog or fast walk and then to a slow walk. You should cool down for at least five to ten minutes, even longer if you're new to exercise.

Muscle Up!

Aerobic exercises don't necessarily strengthen your muscles or increase their size. You already know how important that is because the more muscle you have, the better you burn calories. The way to build more muscle and stronger muscle is through strength training with exercise machines, free weights, elastic resistance bands, and strength-building exercises.

You have a lot of different muscles, but when you exercise, you're basically targeting six major muscle groups:

Shoulders	Upper back
Arms	Chest
Trunk	Legs and buttocks

Different exercises work out different muscle groups. For example, squats and lunges strengthen your legs and butt, whereas abdominal crunches strengthen your trunk or midsection. Push-ups work your chest, and rowing exercises strengthen your upper back. Your goal is to exercise each muscle group at least twice a week. You should always warm up before strength training and cool down afterward, just as you do for aerobic exercise. Because muscles are actually pulled and damaged slightly during weight training, skip a day for rest and healing between sessions.

Whether you join a gym or do your muscle work at home, here's where it really pays to hire a personal trainer to teach you proper form and safe procedures. Even if you buy a great guide and follow written exercise instructions to a "T," you might not be getting the full benefits of your exercises, and you could be hurting yourself without realizing it. If you work out at home, try to find a certified trainer through a local gym. You can also call one of the following organizations for a referral to someone in your area:

American Council on Exercise
(800) 825-3636

Aerobics and Fitness Association of America
(800) YOUR BODY
(800) 968-7263

How Strong Are You?

Your muscle strength and endurance will improve over time if you do strengthening exercises, just as your aerobic capacity improves by doing aerobic exercise. It helps your motivation to keep track of your progress so you can measure improvements. To monitor your upper- and lower-body strength, try these exercises and track your progress once a month:

1. To test your upper-body strength, do as many complete push-ups as you can. Try for at least eight to ten at first. You can go straight for full military-style push-ups, with your legs fully extended, but some people prefer to begin with the type of push-up pictured here.

Testing your upper-body strength with push-ups.

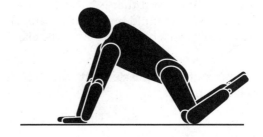

2. To test your lower-body strength, use "wall sits." Lean your back against a solid wall and bend your legs as shown in the figure. Memphis-based exercise physiologist Angela Redden calls these "90 for 90" because the ultimate goal she establishes for clients is 90 degree sits for 90 seconds. Until you get to that point, however, hold the position at a comfortable angle as long as you can. Redden even suggests starting off with three to five sets lasting ten seconds each.

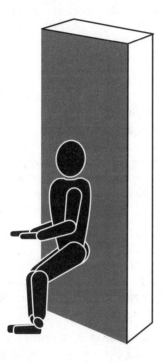

Testing your lower-body strength with "wall sits."

Track your monthly performance at these strength tests on the Strength Log below (make as many photocopies of the log as you need).

Strength Log

	Date:	Date:	Date:	Date:
Upper Body No. of Pushups				
Lower Body Time				

Cross-Training

Cross-training simply means adding a variety of exercises to your workout routine, instead of sticking to just one or two. It means choosing different aerobic exercises, lifting weights, and using other types of strength training and flexibility exercises to get fit. Other names for cross-training routines are circuit training, intervals, and rotations. When you cross-train, you use different muscles, bones, and joints for different exercises, so your whole body gets a good workout and there's less chance you'll damage any one body part by overuse. If you cross-train, you're less likely to get bored, and that's very important when you're trying to stay motivated.

Most professional trainers recommend aerobic exercise at least three or four times a week, alternating with two to three days of strength training. That type of schedule is a form of cross-training in itself. You can also cross-train by doing different exercises on different days. Ride your bike one day, take a dance class the next, and go for a swim the day after that. Of course, you can do more than one type of exercise in a day. Ride your bike to the pool or to the dance class!

Another way to approach cross-training is to combine indoor and outdoor activities. You might work out with free weights and resistance bands in your living room and then move outdoors to run. If you own a treadmill, you might do your running indoors and play tennis or handball at an outdoor court.

Table 17.1 gives examples of common exercises. Use it to mix and match a cross-training program of your own. One from column A and one from column B and… you get the picture!

NutriTip
The average exerciser doesn't get any benefit from dietary supplements or protein powders packaged as performance enhancers and muscle builders. What you need for a good workout is a balanced diet that provides more than half your calories from carbohydrates. Carbohydrates fuel exercise better than any other nutrient.

No Weigh!
Don't limit yourself to only one or two types of exercise. To keep your whole body conditioned and keep your workout from getting boring, vary the type of exercise you do from day to day, and as you get more fit, add new types of workouts to your routine.

Table 17.1 Common Types of Exercises

Aerobic	Muscle Strength and Endurance	Flexibility
Fast walking	Free weights	Yoga
Jogging	Machine weights	Stretches
Swimming	Sit-ups	T'ai chi
Bicycling	Pull-ups	
In-line skating	Push-ups	
Basketball	Body-shaping classes	
Cross-country skiing		
Dance aerobic classes		

Walk This Way

Some people make a real sport out of walking. When I jog around the park in my neighborhood, I often see a woman who walks briskly and boxes with an invisible partner at the same time. I also see a woman walking and doing t'ai chi moves at the same time. Of course, I live in New York City, where you can do these things in public and no one thinks twice about it! Walking is great because you already know how to do it. You don't need a class or a personal trainer to show you how. It's an easy way to start a fitness program.

If walking is one of your primary ways to get exercise, you should have a routine and a plan, just as you would with any other exercise program. Walking is something you can do every day. Pick a time—early morning, during your lunch break, or early evening after dinner—and stick to it. Warm up with a slow walk and work into a brisk walk. Cool down with more slow walking. Aim to increase the amount of time you spend walking quickly as well as the distance you go. Keep track of your distance and timing so you can monitor your progress.

No Weigh!
Don't skimp when it comes to walking shoes. If you walk a lot for exercise, go to an athletic shoe store and choose an appropriate sneaker or walking shoe. Be sure it fits properly, provides good support, and feels comfortable. If you have to make a choice, go for substance over style.

To keep walking interesting, wear a cassette, radio, or CD headphone and switch music often. Pick up a copy of *Walking* magazine for tips and ideas to enhance your routine.

Walk in different directions and on different types of terrain. Search out hills and slopes in your neighborhood. Take hikes in other areas and go on walking vacations. Here's a great idea for adventure walking: A group in Washington, D.C., keeps track of old railroad tracks that have been converted to trails. More than 900 of these trails have been established throughout the United States, covering almost 10,000 miles, and all of them are suitable for walking. For more information on where these trails are and how to walk them, contact

Rails-to-Trails Conservancy
1100 17th St., NW, 10th Floor
Washington, DC 20036
(202) 331-9696
Web site address: www.railtrails.org

Your Walking Style

Believe it or not, there's a proper way to walk and it's possible you've been doing it wrong your whole life! Hint: You're not supposed to slouch! That's right. Walk tall and proud with your shoulders back and your head held high. If you walk long distances and you're not doing it correctly, you can cause yourself a great deal of discomfort. That will eventually slow you down. When you're walking to improve your fitness, you can walk more quickly than usual and keep your arms bent at the elbows, but it's not necessary to take longer strides or make any exaggerated movements.

Walking Off Calories

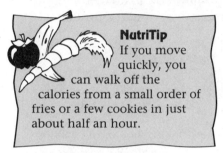

NutriTip
If you move quickly, you can walk off the calories from a small order of fries or a few cookies in just about half an hour.

Obviously, the faster you walk, the more calories you'll burn in a given period of time. Some walkers start off slow and walk at a normal pace for five or ten minutes and then speed up to a brisk walk. You can speed up and slow down for 10- or 15-minute intervals to keep walking interesting and over time, you should be able to walk longer at a higher speed. If you're new to fitness walking, aim for a 15-minute mile. Walking uphill takes more work (and therefore burns more calories) than walking on a straight path. It also helps you work different muscles.

Keeping Track

Whether you're focused on walking or running, going to a gym, or mixing it up by cross-training, you'll stay more motivated if you have real evidence (both on paper and on your bod) of the fruits of your labor. Record your progress on the Exercise Log on the following page. Make extra copies so you have plenty of logs on hand. You can also use a copy of the log as a planner to develop an exercise schedule in advance. Even if you're starting with just a walk around the block, write it down. Next to the day of the week, fill in the exercise you did, the type of exercise it was, and the amount of time you spent doing it. If you exercise regularly, you'll see improvement in your timing and pacing within a few weeks, and your logs will become part of your motivation to keep going.

Exercise Log

Day/Date	Exercise	Category (i.e. aerobic or strength)	Time
Monday	_____	_____	_____
	_____	_____	_____
	_____	_____	_____
Tuesday	_____	_____	_____
	_____	_____	_____
	_____	_____	_____
Wednesday	_____	_____	_____
	_____	_____	_____
	_____	_____	_____
Thursday	_____	_____	_____
	_____	_____	_____
	_____	_____	_____
Friday	_____	_____	_____
	_____	_____	_____
	_____	_____	_____
Saturday	_____	_____	_____
	_____	_____	_____
	_____	_____	_____
Sunday	_____	_____	_____
	_____	_____	_____
	_____	_____	_____

The Least You Need to Know

➤ Aerobic exercise conditions your heart if you exercise within your training heart rate range for at least 20 minutes, three times a week.

➤ Strength training to build more and stronger muscle is just as important to fitness and weight control as any aerobic activity.

➤ The ideal approach to exercise is cross-training, which combines a variety of aerobic activities with a variety of strength-training and flexibility exercises.

➤ If you do it often enough, long enough, and fast enough, you can walk your way to a healthy weight.

Part 6
Mind Over Matter

This part of the book is different from the other parts. The chapters here don't have much to do with food or exercise, but they have everything to do with losing weight.

If you eat in response to your emotions, this part is for you. If you often eat when you're not hungry, there's something here for you, too. These next three chapters provide tools you can use to identify and eliminate all the eating triggers in your life that have nothing to do with real hunger. Some of these triggers come from inside of you and some from outside, but they all need to be addressed before you can move on and get to a healthy weight.

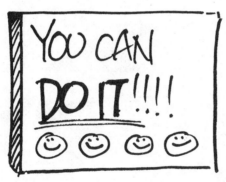

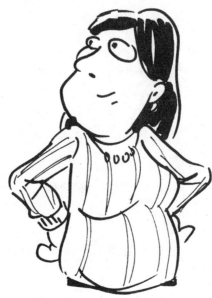

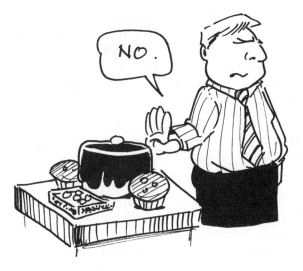

Chapter 18

Changing Your Ways

In This Chapter

➤ Making a commitment to yourself

➤ Are you eating because you're hungry?

➤ Out with your old eating habits, in with the new

➤ How to change your attitude

It's not bad food that makes you fat; it's bad habits. Changing bad habits into good ones is a tough job. Most people resist any kind of change, even when it's for the better. We like to keep things familiar. That's why change is usually slow-going.

Successful weight loss is about slowly changing your behavior. If you speed up the process, you're likely to give up before you reach your goals. Too much change, too soon, is disturbing for most people. When it comes to changing lifestyle habits, too much too soon can be downright overwhelming. This chapter helps you identify habits that need changing and suggests steps you can take right now to get the process started—slowly.

Promises, Promises

If you've been yo-yo dieting most of your life and your weight's gone up and down as a result, you might be afraid to make another commitment to losing weight. Instead of promising yourself you'll lose weight, promise you'll start taking better care of yourself by eating healthier foods and getting more exercise. Losing weight will be the extra bonus you get for healthy living.

No Weigh!
Don't be afraid to try to develop healthier habits and lose weight now just because you've been unsuccessful in the past. It's another time, you're at another stage in your life, and you might be more prepared to make the necessary commitment.

Losing weight doesn't have to be an all-or-nothing proposition. A lot of people make the mistake of losing faith in themselves and giving up after one indulgence. You haven't blown anything with one meal or one dessert or even one all-out binge. Tomorrow's a new day, as they say, and you can pick up your healthy eating habits again just where you left off.

You know you have enough motivation to get started, but what you need now is a firm commitment to see yourself through times of change. You're accustomed to eating a certain amount of food at certain times. You have eating habits that are strongly ingrained. If you need to lose a substantial amount of weight, you're probably talking about changing lifelong habits. You've probably had the habits longer than you've carried the extra weight. Even if you're just trying to shake off ten pounds, you still have to be committed to making changes in your diet and exercise habits.

Commitment means you're not going to give up on yourself. You're going to keep at it until your new eating and exercise habits become just that, habits. You will stick with it until you get to the point where you're more motivated to move forward than backward.

Make a commitment to good health, not just to losing pounds or wearing a particular pants size. That way, you'll be less likely to fall for diet gimmicks that don't work. You won't be so tempted to try yet another fad diet. You'll realize all those "magic bullet" solutions only get in the way of real progress because they distract you from getting to the root of your weight problem. You can do it. You can say to yourself right now, "I'm going to be a healthy person and I'm not going to let anything get in my way." Period.

Guru's Corner
"If you're eating spontaneously when you're not even hungry, you're indulging in immediate gratification. You don't stop that by denying yourself gratification from food. Instead, practice *delaying* gratification. There's always something else you could do besides eat. Go tweeze your eyebrows or trim a hedge. Put off eating and do something constructive at the same time."

—Laurie Deutsch Mozian, M.S., R.D., Nutrition Counselor, Woodstock, New York

Are You Hungry?

Sometimes we eat to satisfy hunger and sometimes we eat to satisfy our appetites. When you feel hunger, you feel a physical need to eat. Your brain acts as a "control center" for hunger so that your body knows when it needs to eat and how much to eat. If you only ate when you were actually hungry, you might not need to lose weight.

Some people don't even know what it's like to be hungry because they've never let themselves feel it. It's important to know what hunger feels like so you can start learning how to eat only in response to the real thing. If you normally eat more often than every three or four hours, try this exercise. Spend a full day paying attention to hunger.

Every time you get up to eat, check your hunger score. On a scale of one to ten, with one being not hungry and ten being ravenously hungry, how hungry are you? If you score five or less, drink a glass of water instead of eating and go back to whatever else you were doing. This type of exercise can help you break a cycle of endless eating. However, don't take it to extremes and avoid eating when you're really hungry. That's self-defeating and will ultimately result in overeating.

How's Your Appetite?

You might not understand your appetite. Your appetite is your *desire* for specific types of food. It's a psychological, rather than physical, need to eat. Your appetite is what's at work when someone puts chocolate mousse or pie à la mode in front of you and you wolf it right down, even though you've just finished a big dinner and you're actually full. In this case, your appetite allows you to eat for sheer pleasure, rather than to satisfy hunger.

When food arouses memories or emotions, you might want to eat even though you're not really hungry. It doesn't matter whether it's a good or bad memory or a positive or negative emotion. If it triggers your appetite and you don't recognize or acknowledge the trigger for what it is, you'll eat. If you have an alternate plan ready, however, you might not eat. The first step is to identify trigger situations and try to eliminate them. Do any of these common trigger situations sound familiar?

> **NutriTip**
> There's a difference between hunger and appetite. Hunger is a physiological need for food. Appetite is a desire for food. When you're trying to lose weight, it helps to know the difference and learn how to eat only when you're truly hungry.

➤ You have a fight with a parent, a sibling, or a spouse.

➤ Someone criticizes you.

➤ You're treated rudely by a sales clerk.

➤ You fear losing a job.

➤ You have a conflict with your boss or a coworker.

➤ You're up against an unrealistic deadline.

➤ Someone cancels a date with you.

➤ You have to do something you dread doing.

Emotional Appetites

You can help yourself break emotional eating habits if you pay attention to triggers and take steps to resist them. Here's why: When you routinely eat three meals a day, at pretty much the same time every day, your body becomes conditioned to expect food at those same times day after day. You start feeling hungry around the time you normally eat breakfast, lunch, and dinner. When you start putting food in your mouth 6, 12, or 20 times a day, your body will start thinking it's hungry all the time, and you'll start feeding it more often. That's how eating gets out of hand for many people. It's hard *not* to eat when you feel the physical sensation of hunger.

Advice from Losers

"When I was an emotional eater, I ate with every emotion. I ate when I was happy, when I was irritated, and when I was bored. I even ate when I was feeling really bad about being fat. Identifying your triggers is a big part of overcoming the problem, but if you can't control it or don't care at the time, knowing won't do you a lot of good. You'll still stuff your face until you get over it. You have to know your solutions and be armed with them. The trick is to figure out exactly what works for you. I head for the gym now, instead of heading for the refrigerator."

—Kelly J.

If you're an emotional eater, your goal is to wait for actual internal signs of hunger before eating, rather than eat in response to outside forces such as stress or anger. If you eat when you're in a distressed or excited state of mind, you're not paying attention to what you're eating or how much you're eating. Here are some alternative behaviors you can try when you know you're not hungry but you're still tempted to eat in response to emotional stress:

➤ Deal with the emotion head on. Express yourself in words rather than in food. If it's not something you feel you can say out loud, write it down.

➤ Go in the opposite direction of any nearby food and stay there for a few minutes to see if the temptation to eat goes away. It just might!

➤ Write your feelings down in a journal.

➤ Set a timer and wait ten minutes.

➤ Go outside for a brisk walk or a run around the block.

➤ Go out and rent a video or buy a magazine.

➤ Repeat after me: Food is *not* the solution.

On the following page is an Alternate Activities Record. It's a little like a food diary except it's designed to help you pay attention to emotional eating and break your pattern of eating when you're not really hungry by choosing a non-food activity instead. Make copies so you'll have one at work, one at home, and one to carry with you when you're on the move. You'll probably have to come up with different activities for different situations. For instance, you might not be able to call a friend when you're bored at work and tempted to eat. In this case, you might choose a work-related task such as updating your Rolodex as your alternate activity.

Alternate Activities Record

Step 1. List ten non-food–related activities you enjoy or can use to delay eating:

1. _____
2. _____
3. _____
4. _____
5. _____
6. _____
7. _____
8. _____
9. _____
10. _____

Step 2. Write down the date, eating cue (hunger, anxiety, saw a picture of food, and so on), and your response. Check eating if you ate in response to the cue, or write down the alternate activity you chose instead. For example:

Date	Eating Cue	Eating	Alternate Activity
7/23	Snack machine	X	
7/23	TV commercial		Brushed teeth
7/23	Lonely		Called Elizabeth

Date	Eating Cue	Eating	Alternate Activity
_____	_____	_____	_____
_____	_____	_____	_____
_____	_____	_____	_____
_____	_____	_____	_____

Know When to Stop

When you eat, your stomach sends a signal to your brain to let it know that food has arrived. Because it takes about 20 minutes for your brain to fully receive the signal that you've had enough food, the time to stop eating is before you feel full. It's also a good reason to eat slowly. When you eat too fast, your stomach fills up before your brain knows you're full, and you end up eating too much food.

> **No Weigh!**
> Don't ignore hunger. If you skip meals because you're too busy to eat or you're trying to avoid eating, you'll just overeat when you finally have a meal.

If you eat a complete meal and leave the table feeling fully satisfied, you're less likely to be hungry and look for more food within the next few hours. A balanced meal—one that contains mostly carbohydrates, some protein, and a little bit of fat—does the best job of keeping you full. That's because different types of foods are digested and absorbed at different rates

Old Habits Die Hard

You might keep slipping into old, familiar habits simply because it's so easy to forget that you're trying to develop new ones. Because I'm a big list keeper, I actually carry written reminders of ways that I want to change. I write down ways I want to be, and the things I need to do to be that way. I carry the note or list around in my wallet in the same section as my money, where I know I'll come across it often. I read it again and again until the new habits take hold. It works if you do it, I promise!

You can also ask other people to remind you about habits you want to break. When I first met this one young friend of mine, she was always saying, "I'm so stupid." I got sick of hearing it pretty quickly, so I called her on it. "I didn't think you were stupid, but you keep saying it, so maybe you're right," I said. I think she was shocked that someone she hardly knew would say that to her, but she asked me to keep doing it. She knew it was a bad habit and wanted to stop, but she was very busy with her life and kept forgetting to work on it. Within a week, she stopped and I haven't heard her slip even once. If you can find people on the job or at home who will remind you that you don't want to eat certain foods or that you're slipping back into an old, destructive routine, such as putting yourself down, take advantage of those people. They could play a big role in your success.

Modified Behavior

There are also plenty of practical ways to change your behavior and break bad eating habits. When you take real-life steps to change the way you respond to eating cues, it's called behavior modification. For example, if you pull up to a soft-serve ice cream stand whenever you drive by it, the stand itself is an eating cue for you. If you take another route so that you don't drive past the stand, you're modifying your behavior to avoid the cue. Some obesity experts think behavior modification is one of most successful techniques for helping people lose weight. Following are some "dos" and "don'ts" to help you avoid or eliminate triggers for overeating:

➤ Don't shop for food when you're hungry.

➤ Do make a shopping list before you go to the grocery store.

➤ Do stick to your shopping list.

➤ Don't buy problem foods, such as snack foods.

➤ Do make a routine out of eating. As often as you can, eat in the same place at the same time.

➤ Do use smaller plates so that your food portions look larger. That way you won't feel short-changed if you're used to eating large portions.

➤ Don't put serving bowls of food on the table. Dish food out on individual plates.

➤ Do leave the table when you've finished eating.

➤ Do encourage family and friends to eat healthier foods with you.

➤ Don't skip meals.

➤ Do keep healthier foods on hand and store them up front in your cupboards and refrigerator.

➤ Do prepare single portions of food when you're cooking just for yourself.

Gura's Corner
"Behavior modification is definitely a means to weight control, but it isn't a unique method in and of itself. It means nothing more than the steps you take to adopt a healthier lifestyle: improving your eating habits and increasing your physical activity."

—Dr. Albert Stunkard; Founder, Weight & Eating Disorders Program; University of Pennsylvania

Table Manners

Behavior modification is a teaching *and* learning process. When you're losing weight on your own, you're both the teacher and the student. Even if you have help, you have to go over the lessons again and again until your new behavior becomes second nature. Here are some more classic behavior modification techniques you can use to train yourself to eat better at home:

➤ Pick one place to eat, such as the kitchen or dining room table, and eat there whenever you have meals or snacks at home. The purpose of this exercise is to narrow down the places in your home that you associate with food and eating.

➤ Always set a complete table service, including a place mat and a pitcher of water, even if you're eating by yourself. This exercise helps you pay more attention to the fact that you're eating and to treat the food you eat with more respect. Don't eat anything—not even a breadstick—until the setting is complete.

➤ Whenever you eat, don't do anything else. Don't watch television or read a magazine or pay bills or talk on the phone. This exercise helps you focus on what you're eating and how much you're eating. It also helps eliminate some of the activities you may unknowingly associate with food.

➤ Drink a full glass of water when you sit down, before you begin to eat. Drink more water while you eat. This will help you feel fuller without adding calories to the meal.

➤ Use small plates and serve yourself small portions. You can always go back for more. This is a great way to get used to smaller portion sizes. After a while, they'll seem normal.

➤ Eat slowly and put your fork down between every bite. Consciously chew every bit of food. The more slowly you eat, the more likely you are to eat only a reasonable amount of food and to recognize when you're full.

Check Your Attitude

No Weigh!
You won't get anywhere with a negative attitude about yourself or your weight-loss goals. To get to a healthy weight, you have to believe you can do it, and you have to believe it's worth doing.

One thing's for sure: You need a can-do attitude to lose weight. If you're having a problem with negative feelings about yourself, try visualization techniques. Visualize yourself where you want to be, not where you are right now. Get a really clear picture of your future self in your mind and hold it there. You need that picture for motivation. It's like a reward dangling almost within your reach. *Believe* in that picture. You're teaching yourself to think forward and look forward, rather than backward, and that's what developing a positive attitude is all about. If you're having a hard time turning your thoughts around, it might help to reread Chapter 4, "Heavy Thoughts."

Change Your Food Attitude

Do you avoid foods you crave because you're afraid you'll eat too much? You may have noticed that the more you tell yourself you can't have a particular food, the more obsessed you become with that food and the more you crave it. So what happens? Sooner or later, you give in and you go overboard. Then what? You probably feel guilty, avoid the food, and start the cycle all over again. What would happen if you just let yourself eat what you like? If you ate a few cookies every day, would that amount to more than what you eat when you finally give in to a desperate craving? Probably not. If you tend to deprive yourself and then overeat, try this: Instead of avoiding indulgence foods, earn them.

➤ Walk to the store to buy a single serving.

➤ Stretch your workout an extra ten minutes.

➤ Save some calories if you know you'll be going out later in the day or that night. Don't skip meals during the day; just eat a little less at each meal so you have some extra calories to play with.

➤ Have a plan. Work small portions of your favorite foods into the day's eating plan.

Have Patience

Patience is another word for inner strength, and sometimes getting to a healthy weight takes a lot of it! It takes a long time to learn new habits, and it's likely you'll have setbacks along the way. Short-term goals are useful when you're feeling impatient with the process of losing weight. Setting a goal just for today or for this week and meeting it will give you a sense that something's happening. You've *done* something about your weight rather than just wait to reach your long-term weight goal.

There are no quick fixes if what you really want is to get to a healthy weight and stay there. That's why it's such an achievement. Many small accomplishments along the way are going to add up to the big one. Rather than get discouraged or impatient because your weight is coming off slowly, celebrate every change you make and every pound you lose because you're that much closer to success.

> **NutriTip**
> As you gradually make the lifestyle changes that are necessary for losing weight, you're also developing the patience you'll need to hang in there until you reach your long-term goal of getting to a healthy weight.

The Least You Need to Know

➤ To lose weight, you have to make a strong commitment to your own good health.

➤ It's important to learn the difference between hunger and appetite. When you feed hunger, you're fulfilling a basic physiological need. When you feed your appetite, you're feeding desires.

➤ One good way to develop new eating habits is to avoid or eliminate the situations that trigger your overeating.

➤ Nothing helps to guarantee successful weight loss more than a positive attitude toward yourself and your future.

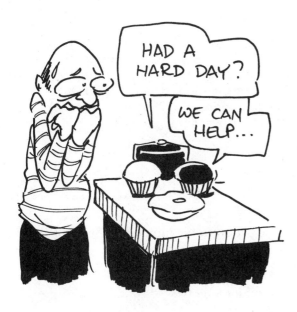

Chapter 19

Handling Your Emotions

In This Chapter

➤ How to figure out whether you're a compulsive overeater

➤ What to do about a negative body image

➤ How excuses and procrastination work against you

➤ Ways to boost your own self-esteem

➤ Stress-busting strategies

Are you looking for love in a cereal box? Psychotherapists say some people use food to diffuse their emotions and block out other problems in their lives by getting lost in eating binges. Sound familiar? If so, this chapter might help you address some of the problems that underlie your overeating.

Are You a Compulsive Overeater?

The dictionary defines compulsion as an irresistible, repeated, irrational impulse to perform some act. If you have an irresistible, repeated, irrational impulse to eat, does that mean you're a compulsive overeater? It might.

Take This Test

According to the folks at Overeaters Anonymous, it isn't only how much you eat that determines the answer, but it's also the way in which you try to control your food. They say if you answer yes to three or more of the following questions (from "Fifteen Questions," Copyright 1986 Overeaters Anonymous, Inc., reprinted with permission of OA, Inc.), you may have or be on your way to a compulsive overeating problem:

1. Do you eat when you're not hungry?
2. Do you go on eating binges for no apparent reason?
3. Do you have feelings of guilt and remorse after eating?
4. Do you give too much time and thought to food?
5. Do you look forward with pleasure and anticipation to the moments when you can eat alone?
6. Do you plan these secret binges ahead of time?
7. Do you eat sensibly before others and make up for it alone?
8. Is your weight affecting the way you live your life?
9. Have you tried to diet for a week (or longer), only to fall short of your goal?
10. Do you resent others telling you to "use a little willpower" to stop overeating?
11. Despite evidence to the contrary, have you continued to assert that you can diet "on your own" whenever you wish?
12. Do you crave to eat at a definite time, day or night, other than mealtime?
13. Do you eat to escape from worries or trouble?
14. Have you ever been treated for obesity or a food-related condition?
15. Does your eating behavior make you or others unhappy?

Dealing with Compulsive Overeating

A number of books have been written about compulsive overeating and emotional overeating, some by trained psychotherapists and some by people who have suffered from the problem themselves. These books are available in regular bookstores and in specialty book shops that carry materials from 12-step recovery programs and their members. (For the names of some books that deal specifically with emotional eating and compulsive overeating, see Appendix B, "Your Best Resources.") One thing these books all seem to have in common is an openness about the underlying emotional and psychological problems associated with compulsive overeating and other eating disorders. If you have an eating disorder or feel you suffer from compulsive overeating, it doesn't mean the problem is all in your head or that if it is indeed in your head, it isn't real.

Advice from Losers

"I've had many stressful problems in my life, and instead of facing them, I spent many years numbing the pain with food. So of course I got very heavy. I started looking high and low for a magic weight-loss solution and spent thousands of dollars getting lost in a lot of other people's diet dreams. But now I know that I was really looking for a quick and easy solution to my problems. I'm no longer a compulsive overeater, just someone trying to lose weight. What works for me now is lots of exercise, watching the amount of fat I eat, and holding on to my own dream of someday helping others get their health back."

—Denise S.

The problems that surface when people talk about compulsive overeating include high stress levels, low self-esteem, and eating in response to anger, confusion, sadness, depression, loneliness, and other emotions. Although there are no clear-cut solutions for compulsive overeaters, it does seem clear that the first step to overcoming compulsive overeating is identifying and understanding all the reasons you eat that have nothing to do with hunger.

Nobody's Perfect

We all make mistakes, but perfectionists don't forgive mistakes. Rather, they tend to judge harshly. If you're a perfectionist, you don't forgive yourself when you make a mistake and you have a hard time forgiving others. Your expectations of yourself and others is unrealistically high. Sometimes, in your search for perfection, you hold some people in too high regard. That only makes it easier for them to disappoint you because your expectations of them are unrealistic. Perfectionism puts quite a strain on your relationship with yourself and everyone else.

If you're a perfectionist, you're probably setting weight-loss goals for yourself that are impossibly high. All you're doing by setting impossible goals is setting yourself up for failure. Instead, set yourself up for success. Learn to accept that your best weight and body shape may be a little less perfect than you think it should be. Just think: If you allow yourself to be just a rung below perfect, you might actually reach your goal! The thrill of reaching an attainable goal sure beats the frustration of never getting to an impossible one.

One of the best things you can do for yourself is switch your focus from the size of your body to the health of your body. Remember that you're a whole person, not just a collection of individual body parts. Think holistically. Pay attention to your whole body, not just your thighs or your abdomen or your chest or whatever part is making you unhappy.

> **No Weigh!**
> Don't think you'll like yourself better or that all your problems will go away after you lose weight. Losing weight only changes your looks, and you might never be content if you depend on your looks for happiness.

In some weight-loss circles, there's a lot of talk about self-love and learning to like yourself before you can lose weight. It's easy to see why self-love can help you get to a healthy weight and stay there. When you love someone, you naturally want to treat that person with care and respect. You don't want to pick that person apart and find fault. You want only the best for that person. When you love *yourself*, it's the same thing. You want to treat yourself better. You want only the best for your body. When you want yourself to have a healthier body, all those lifestyle changes you need to make become easier to accomplish.

Instead of thinking of yourself as fat, think of yourself as out of balance. You've been eating an unbalanced diet or you haven't been balancing the food you eat with an equal amount of exercise—or both. Once your lifestyle becomes balanced, however, so will your body. You *will* reach and maintain a healthy weight!

Excuses, Excuses

You say you want to lose weight and get fit, but you're not doing it. Why not? Can't find the motivation? Afraid you won't get it right? Don't have the time? Sorry, but you can, you will, and you do. And you know it.

Putting It Off

You probably find time for most of the things you want to do—that is, the things you *really* want to do. If you're hungry, you always find time to eat. Why can't you find the time to eat right? If you're a workaholic, you always find time for work. But when it comes to exercise, you can't seem to squeeze it in.

If you're putting off losing weight because the whole idea seems so huge, relax. Even though this is a big book about losing weight, it doesn't present a big, overwhelming challenge. Getting to a healthy weight is a slow, deliberate process. (I recently heard a good joke about this: If you think time flies, get on a treadmill!)

> **NutriTip**
> If you look at change as an adventure or opportunity, rather than something you're forced to do, you'll have a more positive attitude about developing new food and exercise habits.

You might procrastinate because you're in a "diet" frame of mind, and you're putting off another attempt to lose weight because deep down, you don't believe it will work. You're procrastinating to avoid another failure.

Procrastination keeps you in a constant state of high anxiety because you're always thinking about something that needs to get done, but you're never doing anything about it. It is probably a whole lot easier to just do the thing than it is to procrastinate about it! When you procrastinate, you stand still. Standing still won't help you get to a healthy weight, that's for sure! Losing weight takes movement.

One way to work toward your goals and procrastinate at the same time is to practice what I call constructive procrastination. If you can't get yourself to do the actual thing it takes to get the job done, do a related thing. That means if you're not ready to join a health club, read about different types of exercise. If you do belong to a health club but can't force yourself to go, get down on the floor and do some push-ups. Warm yourself up and do some stretches. Just be sure to do *something* related to your goal. This book is full of ideas—big and small—for keeping yourself on the path to a healthy weight. Here are a few more:

➤ Get a massage to reduce stress. It's better to stop off at a spa on the way home from work than a doughnut shop.

➤ Join in a jump-rope marathon with your kid. This is not a competition, just a way to exercise and have fun with your child at the same time.

➤ Buy a Japanese cookbook. This cuisine is naturally low in fat.

➤ Take a class in anatomy and physiology. Learn how your body works.

Pointing Your Finger

No one likes to be blamed or held completely responsible for a bad outcome. Are you a blamer? Take this mock-quiz and find out! (Circle the correct answer.)

Who's fault is it that you're fat?

(a) Your boss, for yelling at you.

(b) Your grandmother, for handing down her genes.

(c) Yours, for overeating.

(d) All of the above.

(e) None of the above.

It may be true that your boss is a maniac, your grandmother passed along her hippo hips, and you have a tendency to drown your sorrows in large bowls of butterscotch pudding. But the correct answer is (e). It's no one's fault that you're fat. You're overweight because of a combination of factors, some of which you can control and some of which you can't. However, you can *deal* with all of them and get to a healthier weight.

Blaming is just another way to avoid losing weight and taking responsibility for your own health. Even when you're pointing the finger in your own

No Weigh!
Don't blame yourself or anyone else for your weight problems. Blame doesn't motivate you to lose weight. It's just something you use as an excuse to avoid the responsibilities that go hand-in-hand with getting healthy.

direction, you're using yourself as an excuse. Think about how much time and energy you spend reinforcing those negative beliefs. Then think of all the different ways that same time could be better spent. Do this: Instead of blaming, try conquering. Instead of giving in and then saying "I ate those peanut butter crackers because I hate my boss," say, "I won't let him get to me this way." Instead of looking at your hips and thinking it's hopeless because you're becoming a dead ringer for your grandmother, *use* the information you have about your genes. Do what you can to prevent your body from getting more and more out of shape.

Self-Esteem

What did you do today? Did you accomplish the things you wanted to accomplish? Did you learn something new? Did you take steps toward reaching your healthy weight? Any positive, forward-moving step you take on any day can help boost your self-esteem. It's hard to feel bad about yourself when you look back over your day, and say in a positive way, "Wow, look what I've done!" It's a great boost to your self-esteem to look back and see some accomplishments.

Stop right now and think about your day—not about what went wrong with it, but what went right with it. Did you laugh about anything? Write down anything you can remember about your day that was an accomplishment, no matter how small or ordinary and no matter what it was about. Here are some examples. If any apply, check them off. Then fill in the blanks at the end with your own personal successes.

- ❑ I walked somewhere instead of driving.
- ❑ I bought a new book.
- ❑ I paid some bills.
- ❑ I bought fruit for dessert.
- ❑ I cleaned the living room.
- ❑ I walked right by the snack machine without buying anything.
- ❑ I signed up for a computer class.
- ❑ I took on a new responsibility at work.
- ❑ I made a new friend.
- ❑ I connected with an old friend.
- ❑ I received a compliment.
- ❑ I gave a compliment.
- ❑
- ❑
- ❑
- ❑

If you're working on self-esteem issues, this is a good exercise to do on a daily basis. It's especially important on a really bad-hair day, when nothing seems to go right. If you take the time to carefully review the day, it's likely you'll find at least one saving event. You have to stop and take the time to think about it, or that good thing can easily get lost in the muck of negative events.

Lighten Up!

Stress is different for different people. You might rise to a challenge that the next person will go out of her way to avoid. Whether or not a situation is stressful depends on how you respond to it. Even though we think of stress as a negative thing, it isn't always. A little stress can actually be a good motivator because it can signal a need for change in your life and give you the push you need to make that change.

Positive changes such as a job promotion, buying a house, getting married, giving birth, or going away to school can cause stress. That's because *any* type of change brings with it a new set of problems and its own forms of stress. It's the negative emotions and behavior that cause the most worrisome form of stress. If you live with a lot of these emotions and behaviors, you're going to feel stress all the time. How many of these negative stressors are ruling your life?

Anger	Fear
Guilt	Perfectionism
Frustration	Resentment
Procrastination	Overwork
Indecision	Anxiety
Regret	Panic
Worry	Criticism

Name Your Stressor

Some stressors come from within, such as a need for everything (including your body) to be perfect or the self-doubt that prevents you from asking your boss for a raise you deserve. These are the types of stress for which you can take responsibility. Other stressors come from outside yourself. These include such events as deaths, car accidents, job layoffs, and other people's behavior that's out of your control. Internal and external stressors can also be positive. If you respond to stress by overeating, the first thing you need to do is identify your particular stressors, both positive and negative. Think about the specific internal and external stressors that exist in your life right now and write them down:

Internal Stressors

_____

_____

_____

_____

External Stressors

_____

_____

_____

_____

Managing Stress

You probably have automatic responses to stress triggers. Well, once again, you're going to have to make changes if you want to reduce stress, and some of these changes will have to be in the way you respond to situations that cause stress. Other changes might involve taking the time to correct a situation or creating a new situation to replace the old one. I'll give you an example. When two good friends decided to move out of town at the same time, I felt all the usual signs of stress. I got panicky and felt a great deal of apprehension about being left behind. One of these friends was also my running partner, so on top of everything else, I was afraid of losing a big source of motivation to exercise. I was stressed, but I knew that the healthiest way to deal with that stress was to reach out to other friends immediately and find a new running partner. As it turned out, I actually found someone in my neighborhood who was also losing her exercise buddy at the same time, so we hooked up and started running together. I also went back to a health club where I happen to know a few members, and I started calling them to make "gym dates." That's how I got the initial motivation I needed to start working out again.

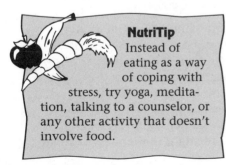

NutriTip
Instead of eating as a way of coping with stress, try yoga, meditation, talking to a counselor, or any other activity that doesn't involve food.

It's not always that easy to manage a stressful situation, but there's always a choice between taking positive and negative steps to ease the symptoms of stress. You know the negative choices: giving up on yourself, overeating, and choosing other self-defeating behavior. Addressing a stressful situation directly is usually the most positive way to handle it. Sometimes you find that all your positive attempts to resolve a situation haven't worked. At that point, the most positive response might be to give up trying to manage the situation and move on. (That's *not* the same as giving up on yourself!)

Take some of the unresolved stressors you listed in the previous section and write down the negative ways you've been responding to them. Then come up with a better or more direct solution. For example:

Stressor	Negative Response	Direct Response
Screaming boss	Self-doubt	Ask for a meeting to discuss problems or look for a new job.
Fight with Mom	Feel guilty	Apologize for yelling and stop trying to control the family.

Stressor	Negative Response	Direct Response
_____	_____	_____
_____	_____	_____
_____	_____	_____
_____	_____	_____

The Least You Need to Know

➤ Compulsive overeaters often struggle with emotional issues that interfere with normal eating patterns.

➤ If you're a perfectionist, you may be setting impossible weight-loss goals for yourself.

➤ Blame and procrastination only serve as excuses for not losing weight.

➤ The happier you are with yourself, the more you'll want to take care of your health.

➤ Once you identify both the positive and negative causes of stress in your life, you can plan other ways to deal with them besides eating.

➤ To attain a healthier weight, you'll need to respond to emotions and stress with something other than food.

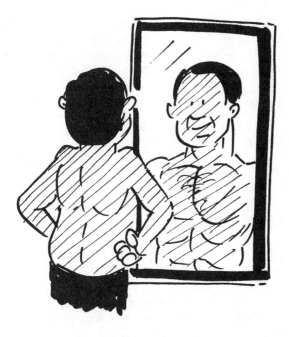

Chapter 20

Thinking Fit

In This Chapter

➤ Finding appropriate role models

➤ Examining your fears

➤ Where to go when you need help

➤ Putting all your tools into practice

Do you know anyone who never diets but always stays in shape? Grab that person and don't let go! Seriously, though, if you want to get fit, you must first learn what it means to *think* fit. Your best teachers are people you can relate to who stay in shape by practicing a positive, healthy lifestyle.

Turn the page to find out what kind of people are most successful at losing weight and how you can get over any fears you have about being one of them.

Who's Your Role Model?

If you've been dreaming an impossible body dream, maybe it's time to get real about your role models. Actors, dancers, athletes, entertainers, supermodels, and even not-so-super models aren't realistic physical role models for most of us. For one thing, they get *paid* to be in near-perfect physical shape. For another, many models, dancers, and other celebrities suffer from anorexia and bulimia. Also, the physical shape you see in a magazine or on-screen has often been "enhanced" to appear more perfect than the person is in real life. It seems like a waste of time to model yourself after an image that was created on a computer or perfected with an air brush—or worse yet, to model yourself after someone who maintains weight with the help of an eating disorder.

Look for everyday people who are trying to live happy, healthy lives. Look for people who are hopeful about themselves and their futures. These are the types of people who can serve as true role models for you. The people I've known who got healthier and lost weight don't give up on themselves, even sometimes after many years of struggling with their weight. Sometimes they survive the ups and downs of life by sheer determination. One of the most successful losers I've ever known has survived 32 surgeries, a couple of divorces, the arrest of a sibling, and the violent death of a parent. She tried diet after diet, and by the time I met her, she knew more about weight loss than I did. Now she's not only successful at maintaining a healthier weight, but also she successfully maintains her can-do attitude. She simply refuses to let life get the best of her. That's a sure sign that someone's on the road to success.

In talking to all kinds of experts for this book as well as many, many people who have struggled with weight for most of their lives, everyone finds that the common thread among the successful is a willingness to do the things they must do to lose and maintain weight. They don't have magic formulas. They exercise, they eat low-fat foods, and they watch how much they eat. They maintain a positive attitude and celebrate their achievements. They find teachers and role models and follow their lead, but they also learn to break rules and individualize their own fitness plans. *They take responsibility for themselves.* They want to be healthy more than they want to do the things that get in the way of that goal. Some say they will never forget the pain of being overweight, and they use that as motivation. If I were to sum up the traits and habits of the successful losers I've known, they would certainly include

➤ Individual determination

➤ Positive attitude

> **Guru's Corner**
> "People who are successful at weight loss don't feel sorry for themselves. Their attitude is that it's worth it to give something up for what they get in return. If you want to lose weight but you also want to eat a lot of food, you'll have to choose one or the other. Ask yourself, 'Which one do I want more?'"
>
> —Anne M. Fletcher, M.S., R.D., author, *Thin for Life* and *Eating Thin for Life* (Houghton Mifflin/Chapters)

> **NutriTip**
> Find people in your own life whom you can use as role models. Find other overeaters who are determined to be successful at getting to a healthy weight. Don't be afraid to copy the ways of people who are doing what you want to do. You won't lose yourself in the process; you'll learn and move on.

➤ Healthy eating habits

➤ Active lifestyles

➤ Honesty

➤ Sense of responsibility

➤ Overall desire to be healthy

➤ Commitment to a healthier lifestyle

No More Fear!

One of the big secrets to losing weight is not being afraid to try. Fear is paralyzing. You can't move forward when you're afraid of the future. Some fears and anxieties are common to the experience of losing weight. What if you lose weight and can't keep it off? What if you lose weight and all your fantasies still don't come true? What if you're hungry all the time? Deep down, you know what to do with your fears. Stand tall and stare them in the face. That's how you desensitize yourself and move forward. It's the only way.

> **No Weigh!**
> Don't let your fears weigh you down like a pair of cement shoes. It doesn't matter whether you fear the frustration of failure or the responsibility of success; you won't be in control of your health until you stare it in the face.

Fear of Fat

I know people who talk about nothing but fat. They're obsessed! I bet you know plenty of people like that, too. If all you think about is fat, however, it sounds like your life is a little out of balance. If you're careful not to get too much fat in your diet, you have a healthy approach to eating. If you worry about the fat in every piece of food you eat, you have a fat phobia. That's no fun! Remember: To stay healthy, you need *some* fat in your diet. If you don't remember why, return to Chapter 11, "You Are What You Eat," and read the section on fat. If you've made a science out of eliminating all fat from your diet, it's time to face your fear. Enjoy an avocado once in a while. Drizzle your salad with a little olive oil. You'll look and feel better for it.

Fear of Success

Believe it or not, even though you say you want to lose weight, you might actually be afraid to do it. You might actually suffer from a fear of getting thin, just like someone who's afraid of professional success. It's not so hard to understand. After all, you've been overweight for a long time, and it's familiar to you. If you lose weight, you'll be looking at a physically new you. You might be afraid of failure. There's always that possibility that you won't lose quite as much weight as you set out to lose. You might fear that once you lose weight, you'll have to live up to some ideal that you're not sure you can live up to.

What if you can't live up to your own ideal of a thinner person? Maintaining a healthy weight can be hard work. Are you afraid to do the work? Don't be afraid to admit it. That's your first step toward success.

Fear of Failure

How many times have you had to learn something "the hard way"? Sometimes you learn your best lessons by doing things wrong the first time, picking yourself up, and trying the same thing again or trying something different. In the language of weight loss, failure is known as a lapse or relapse. You lapse back into an old, destructive habit. You'll probably suffer a lapse or two on your way to a healthy weight. Most people do. There's really only one healthy way to deal with lapses: Allow yourself to "fail," watch yourself get up and get over it, and you won't have anything left to fear.

What Are You Afraid Of?

Before you can face your fears, you have to know what they are. Are you afraid of hunger? Are you afraid of the emotions you're covering up? Copy the Facing Your Fears Worksheet below and write down the things that scare you the most when you think about getting fit and losing weight. Next to your fear, write down at least one way you can think of to face it. That will usually involve participating in the very action you fear. For example, you might be afraid to tell your partner that you're starting a healthy eating program out of fear that the response will be something such as, "Oh no, not again!" You might face that fear by setting up a time to talk about it in the near future.

Facing Your Fears Worksheet

The Fear	The Face-Off
_____	_____
_____	_____
_____	_____
_____	_____
_____	_____
_____	_____

Help Is Here

Losing weight is a personal matter, and everyone has to find his or her own road to success. Along the way, no matter who you are, you'll probably need help. You might have to draw from many different sources to get all the help you need. Never fear, it's out there. Help is all around you in the form of magazine articles, health clubs, counselors, self-help books, Web sites, cooking classes, and support groups. You just have to take the first step and seek help.

To keep things interesting, look for new sources of help and support. If you have a computer and Internet access, you literally have a world of diet and exercise information at your fingertips. Surf the Web, and you'll find weight-loss support groups, health club and exercise information, low-fat recipes, magazine articles, and leads for professional help. The best thing about the Web is the people who contribute to it. It's one thing to get tips from professionals and another to get advice from people who've "been there." You'll find both on the Web. There's plenty of reliable health and nutrition information on the Internet, but be sure to question advice from anyone who has something to sell.

The surest way to control what's in the food you eat is to prepare it yourself. If you don't know how to cook or feel you're stuck in a cooking rut, take a class. If there are no cooking schools in your area, try calling a local university or cooperative extension or even a large hospital. Funny as that might sound, cooking classes designed for people with diabetes and heart disease are actually well suited for anyone who wants to lose weight. That's because the lessons are designed to teach calorie and portion control as well as low-fat cooking and balanced meal planning—everything you need to know about healthful eating!

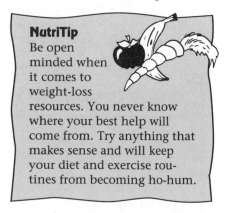

NutriTip
Be open minded when it comes to weight-loss resources. You never know where your best help will come from. Try anything that makes sense and will keep your diet and exercise routines from becoming ho-hum.

Things can get tough when you're working on your weight loss alone. Even if you're determined to do it yourself, you might want to check out a local support group or work with a private counselor for a while, especially if you're trying to lose more than the proverbial ten pounds. It never hurts to have the support of someone who knows what you're going through and who can offer constructive, unbiased advice.

Practice, Practice, Practice

One reason you need patience to successfully lose weight is that you have to practice new habits over and over again until you get them right. That can take time! If you have a lot of weight to lose, you're talking about changing eating, exercising, and thinking habits that have been with you for a long time. Because the best way to learn new habits is one or two at a time, it's going to take a while.

Get Positive

As discussed in Chapter 4, "Heavy Thoughts," self-talk is the conversation you have with yourself that often reflects and determines how you feel about yourself. It takes a great deal of practice for most people to switch from negative self-talk to positive self-talk. The longer you've been thinking damaging thoughts, the more deeply embedded they are in your mind and the longer it can take to get into a habit of replacing them with more productive, positive thoughts. I've seen people work hard to eliminate specific negative references from their vocabulary, only to replace them with a new negative vocabulary.

This is an exercise you might have to pick up again and again while you're trying to lose and maintain weight. Be patient. Turning negative thoughts into positive might be one of the most important steps you take to get to your healthy weight. A positive approach can help you believe that you can lose weight, and once you believe in yourself, nothing can stop you. Study the examples of negative self-talk converted to positive in the Positive Thoughts worksheet below, and then write down your own negative thoughts in the blanks provided. Next to each negative thought, write down a positive replacement thought. Repeat your positive thoughts out loud, again and again, until you're sure you won't forget them. That way, the next time you start to slip into negative thought patterns, your new thoughts will be right there in the front of your mind, ready to fill in.

Positive Thoughts Worksheet

Negative	Positive
I haven't lost enough weight.	This is great. I'm a pound lighter than I was two weeks ago!
I'm going to gain all my weight back.	This binge was just a temporary lapse.
This isn't working.	Good things take time.
I shouldn't eat this food.	I'm going to figure out a way to fit this food into my plan.
I'm not doing as well as I could be doing.	I'm proud of what I've done so far.
_____	_____
_____	_____
_____	_____
_____	_____
_____	_____

That's Affirmative!

Like positive self-talk, an affirmation is an optimistic thought or vision that represents a belief. Affirmations can be spiritual or practical, but they are always encouraging and uplifting. I think of affirmations as gentle, "softening" statements because my attitude softens whenever I read them. Unlike positive self-talk, however, affirmations are optional. They're not absolutely essential for weight loss. In fact, not everyone feels comfortable with affirmations. Some people are uneasy using "touchy-feely" tools and would rather stick to facts and practical solutions for weight control. Like meditation and other relaxation techniques, however, affirmations can help lift some of the "emotional weight" we all carry with us. With a lightened emotional load, it's sometimes easier to deal with the physical task of losing weight.

Advice from Losers

"I'm 39 years old and my journey to recovery began nine years ago. For some of us, recovery from obesity means digging deep down into some painful memories and facing our tormentors. Yes, it takes good nutrition, exercise, and probably some willpower to lose weight. But to anyone who has never battled obesity themselves, I say there is a part of our core you can never understand. My recovery is a work in progress, but there is progress now that I have a special support group that helps me deal with the whole physical and emotional package."

—Barbara S.

Affirmations for Getting to a Healthy Weight

Most affirmations are short phrases or statements, such as "I like myself" or "I am winning the fight." To use an affirmation, you simply have to read it and repeat it to yourself. Many people read affirmations early in the day and again at the end of the day. Some carry their favorite affirmations in their wallets as a reminder. Make up your own affirmations and add them to this list:

➤ I'm getting healthy.

➤ I can lose weight.

➤ I will be successful

➤ I can wait as long as it takes.

➤ I have respect for my body.

➤ I feel positive.

➤ I'm getting there.

➤ I enjoy being healthier.

➤ My life is worth living.

➤ I enjoy my food.

➤ I have choices.

➤ My body is getting stronger.

➤ My diet is becoming more balanced.

➤ I'm reaching my goals.

➤ My life is changing for the better.

➤ I enjoy exercising my body.

➤ I can say no to destructive behavior.

➤ My mind is getting stronger.

➤ I'll get what I want.

➤ I feel peaceful.

➤ I'm proud of myself.

➤ I'm in control of my health.

➤ I can do it.

➤ I'm excited about losing weight.

➤ _____

➤ _____

➤ _____

➤ _____

233

Words for Change

If you like to write, you can use affirmations as a starting point for exploring your own values and beliefs. I like to take affirmations that suggest a trait I don't have but would like to have and explore the ways I could develop that trait. Here's one I wrote recently:

> I am a patient person. I can wait on lines and use the time to complete thoughts that were left hanging earlier in the day. I am a patient person. I can listen until the other person finishes talking. I am a patient person. I can go for hours without looking at my watch.

Unfortunately, none of this is true about me on a day-to-day basis. I'm only patient in certain specific situations. But by being honest in a round-about way and exploring the concept of patience, I see some real possibilities. I see what I need to do to develop more patience. Try exploring the concept of a healthy body in the following exercise. Fill in the blanks with your ideas about what you need to do to have a healthy body.

My body is healthy. _____
_____.

My body is healthy. _____
_____.

My body is healthy. _____
_____.

The Least You Need to Know

➤ Choose realistic role models who trying to live healthy, hopeful lives.

➤ Everyone has fears. Identifying and confronting your fears about losing weight is the first step to getting over them.

➤ Support comes in many different forms, from human to electronic. Be open-minded and you'll find all the help you need.

➤ Developing new eating, exercising, and thinking patterns takes patience and practice.

Part 7
Your Personal Plan for Losing Weight

Keeping track and staying in control of what you eat when you're trying to lose weight is smart. Counting every single calorie and obsessing about every gram of fat in every piece of food you eat is dumb. The following chapters show you how, with a little planning, you can grab a burger or a slice of pizza for lunch, go to parties, eat dessert, and do just about anything you want to do while you're losing weight. Real life doesn't have to get in the way; it just has to be taken into consideration.

In this last part, you'll find three flexible eating plans, a helpful supermarket shopping guide, and a few quick, easy, low-fat recipes and ideas for everyday cooking. You'll see that your eating plan can be any way you want it. And that will be the simple secret of your success.

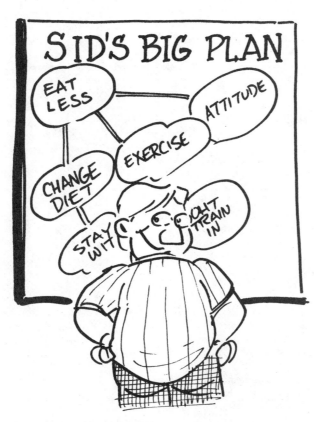

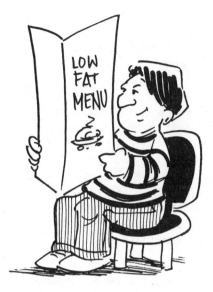

Chapter 21

Your Menu for Weight Loss

In This Chapter

➤ Choosing a healthy eating plan

➤ Menus for weight loss

➤ Eat what you want

➤ Fair exchanges

➤ Living a low-fat life

The problem with most weight-loss diets is that they're just too rigid. You have to eat exactly what and when the diet tells you. The diet is only guaranteed for as long as you stick to it exactly, and that doesn't work for most people. Most people need a little more flexibility from a food plan.

This chapter gives you choices. You can choose from three interchangeable eating plans. Whichever one you choose becomes your personal plan. If you get bored with it, or it doesn't work out for some reason, you can switch to another. The plans are actually quite similar to each other so it's easy to move from one to the other.

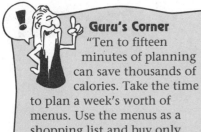

Pick a Plan

There are a number of different ways to approach eating when you're trying to lose weight. Obviously, you have to control the number of calories you consume, no matter which approach you take. That doesn't mean you actually have to *count* calories, unless you want to. Maybe you just want to eat. Here are three plans that let you do just that. Each plan is nutritionally balanced and each provides about 1,500 to 1,600 calories. The only difference is the structure of each plan. Choose the one that's most appealing to you, and I'll help you work out the details later in the chapter. If it becomes inconvenient or boring, you can switch to another plan. In fact, you can switch from plan to plan whenever you like, even from day to day. Here are the three eating plans:

➤ **Straight Menu Plan.** This plan is the most structured and probably the easiest to start with. If you don't want to do any thinking for yourself, this plan's for you. All you have to do is follow the menus as written, and you'll be eating balanced, low-fat, calorie-controlled meals every day. You can also use the menus as guides for designing your own menus, by substituting equal amounts of similar foods at any meal. This is the plan that was introduced in Chapter 10, "Ready, Set Go!" It makes sense for most people because there's enough structure to keep your eating in control, but also enough flexibility to include whatever foods you feel like eating.

➤ **Pick-A-Meal Plan.** This is a variation on the straight menu plan that lets you put together a day's worth of balanced meals by picking foods you like to eat from a mix-and-match menu. Again, you can follow the menus as written or, whenever you like, substitute foods from similar food groups.

➤ **Open Exchange Plan.** This plan is the least structured of the three. There are no menus. As with the flexible menu plans, you must learn to recognize and eat typical serving sizes. Beyond that, you get a specific number of food "exchanges," or servings from each food group, and you use them any way you please. This is a method you can use to keep track of the types and amounts of food you eat when you don't have time to plan meals. However, this plan is too flexible for anyone who wants to learn how to eat regular, balanced meals. If you're trying to control how often you eat, an open exchange probably isn't the right plan for you because it allows you to eat whatever you want and whenever you want throughout the day. There's no formal meal plan in an open exchange system.

Straight Menu Plan

If you want to follow a straight menu plan for healthy eating, use these five menus that follow the plan introduced in Chapter 10. Feel free to make any substitutions you want. Just stick to similar food groups and eat similar amounts of food when you substitute so you keep your meals nutritionally balanced and stay within your calorie range.

Breakfast

1 whole grain bagel

$1/4$ cup "light" ricotta cheese or low-fat cottage cheese

1 kiwi

Lunch

$1^1/2$ cups lentil and ham soup

1 whole-wheat roll

1 ounce of cheese

2 cups spinach and carrot salad with low-fat dressing

Dinner

1 small salmon steak

$1/2$ cup mashed potatoes (made with milk and a little butter)

1 cup green beans with tomatoes

1 slice Italian bread

1 teaspoon butter or margarine

2 poached pear halves

Snack

2 rice cakes topped with

2 tablespoons apple butter

1 cup low-fat milk

Breakfast

$1/4$ cantaloupe melon

1 oat bran muffin

1 cup low-fat milk

Lunch

2 cups mixed green salad with

2 slices avocado and low-fat dressing

$1^1/2$ cups black bean soup

12 low-fat tortilla chips

1 orange

Dinner

1 lamb chop

1 baked potato topped with

$1/2$ cup low-fat plain yogurt

1 cup steamed spinach sprinkled with

1 chopped tomato and

$1/4$ cup crumbled feta cheese

Snack

2 cups low-fat microwave popcorn

$3/4$ cup pineapple juice

Breakfast

1 cup hot cooked cereal such as Wheatena or oatmeal

1 cup low-fat milk

$1/2$ mango

Lunch

1 roast beef sandwich

$^1/_2$ cup baby carrot sticks

1 cup fresh pineapple cubes

Dinner

2 cups cooked pasta with

$^1/_2$ cup tomato sauce mixed with

1 chopped fresh tomato and

$^1/_4$ cup chopped fresh basil topped with

2 Tbsp. grated Parmesan

1 slice Italian bread

1 tsp. butter or margarine

1 cup steamed asparagus

Snack

5 multi-grain crackers

1 oz. cheddar cheese

Breakfast

Banana-berry health shake made in a blender with

1 banana

$^1/_2$ cup fresh or frozen strawberries

1 cup nonfat plain or vanilla yogurt

2 tablespoon nonfat dry milk powder

1 tablespoon wheat germ or bran

2 ice cubes

Lunch

Turkey and tomato sandwich on whole grain bread

$^1/_2$ cup barley or rice and vegetable salad

Dinner

Spinach and orange salad with low-fat dressing

1 cup meat or bean chili

1 small square corn bread

2 pineapple slices

Snack

$1/2$ cup low-fat frozen yogurt

Breakfast

$1/2$ grapefruit

1 English Muffin with

1 scrambled egg and

1 slice lean ham

1 cup low-fat milk

Lunch

1 pita bread filled with

3 falafel and

1 sliced tomato and

$1/2$ cup low-fat, plain yogurt sauce

10 grapes

Dinner

2 cups tofu or meat and broccoli stir-fry

$1/2$ cup cooked rice

2 cups spinach, cucumber, and radish salad with low-fat dressing

Snack

1 cup low-fat milk with 1 Tbsp. chocolate syrup

1 banana

Pick a Meal

The only difference between this approach and a straight menu plan is that you create a daily menu by picking one each from a selection of different breakfast, lunch, and dinner menus.

There are no strict rules about substitutes other than to stay in the same food group when you switch individual foods. To make sure your diet is nutritionally and calorically balanced, it's best to pick one breakfast, one lunch, and one dinner each day (from the columns in the Pick-a-Meal Choices chart), rather than, say, one breakfast, and two lunches. But it's even okay to do that once in a while if it's more convenient. You can also choose a daily snack from the Snack column. To be sure your diet is well balanced, choose different menus and different snacks from day to day.

Pick-a-Meal Choices

Breakfast	Lunch	Dinner	Snack
1 kiwi 2 small pancakes 2 Tbsp. reduced-calorie pancake syrup 1 cup low-fat milk	1 cup vegetable soup 1 roast beef sandwich 1 pear	1 small chicken breast 1 cup steamed green beans 1 cup yellow squash $1/2$ cup cooked couscous 1 tspn. butter or margarine	12 grapes 1 ounce cheese
$1/2$ cup low-fat cottage cheese $1/2$ cup cut-up pineapple 1 toasted English muffin 2 Tbsp. fruit spread	1 cup low-fat yogurt topped with $1/2$ cup fruit salad and 2 tablespoons wheat germ 1 small muffin	1 cup vegetable soup 1 small pork chop $1/4$ cup unsweetened applesauce $1/2$ sweet potato $1/2$ cup sliced zucchini with tomatoes	2 cups reduced-fat popcorn $3/4$ cup grape juice

Breakfast	Lunch	Dinner	Snack
1 small corn muffin 2 slices reduced-fat bacon or 1 ounce lean ham 1 slice melon 1 cup skim milk	1 Chef's Salad 1 small roll or breadstick 2 peach halves 1 cup low-fat milk	2 cups mixed green salad with tomatoes and low-fat dressing 1 broiled fish fillet 1 cup broccoli $1/2$ cup rice 1 tspn. butter or margarine	$1/2$ cup low-fat frozen yogurt with 1 sliced banana
1 cup low-fat yogurt topped with $1/4$ cup low-fat granola 1 banana	1 slice whole-grain toast topped with 2 Tbsp. peanut butter and 2 Tbsp. raisins 1 apple 1 cup low-fat milk	1 cup cooked pasta $1/4$ cup marinara sauce 2 lean turkey sausages 1 tablespoon grated Parmesan 1 thin slice Italian bread $1/2$ cup steamed spinach	$1/2$ cup peach halves with $1/2$ cup low-fat frozen yogurt
$1/2$ grapefruit 2 scrambled eggs 2 slices whole-grain toast 2 Tbsp. fruit spread	1 cheese and tomato sandwich 1 cup fruit salad 1 cup low-fat milk	1 lean hamburger or turkey burger on 1 hamburger roll with Lettuce, tomato, and catsup $1/2$ cup baby carrot sticks $1/2$ cup corn	1 cup low-fat milk with 1 Tbsp. chocolate syrup 1 mini-muffin

Breakfast	Lunch	Dinner	Snack
3/4 cup cereal flakes with 1 cup berries 1 cup low-fat milk	1 cup lentil soup 1 small roll or 4 crackers 2 cups mixed green salad with low-fat dressing 1 cup grapes 1 cup low-fat milk	1 cup egg drop soup 2 cups meat or tofu stir-fry with mixed vegetables 1/2 cup rice	1/4 cup hummus (chick-pea dip) 5 crackers
1 small whole-grain muffin 1/2 cup "light" ricotta cheese with 1 apple	2 cups pasta salad with vegetables 1 breadstick 1 orange	1 spinach and mushroom salad with low-fat dressing 1 enchilada (any kind) 1/2 cup rice 1/2 cup black beans	2 graham crackers 1 cup milk

The Open Exchange Plan

In Chapter 13, "Take a Look at Your Eating Habits," you were introduced to the food groups that make up the Food Guide Pyramid. You learned how many servings of food you should eat from each food group. You also learned the appropriate serving sizes of different foods within each group. On the Open Exchange Plan, you can use the pyramid servings as a guide to what and how much food you should eat. You don't have to plan your meals in advance or follow a ready-made menu. Instead, photocopy and use the 1,600 Calorie Open Exchange Checklist on the following page to keep track of your food throughout each day.

1,600 Calorie Open Exchange Checklist						
6 bread, approx. 480 calories	❑	❑	❑	❑	❑	❑
2 meat/meat alternatives, approx. 300–500 calories	❑	❑				
3 vegetables, approx. 75 calories	❑	❑	❑			
2 fruit, approx. 150 calories	❑	❑				
2–3 milk/dairy, approx. 200–450 calories	❑	❑	❑			
2 added fat (2 teaspoons), approx. 80 calories	❑	❑				

How It Works

As you can see, on a 1,600 calorie eating plan, you get six bread servings, two meat or meat alternative servings, three vegetable servings, two fruit servings, and two to three milk/dairy servings. You're also allowed two teaspoons of added fat for the day. That helps you account for any added butter, margarine, vegetable oil, mayonnaise, or cream cheese you use. If you used low-fat versions of these products, you can stretch those two teaspoons to a tablespoon.

Even though this is a 1,600 calorie plan, you can see on the 1,600 Calorie Open Exchange Checklist that your actual calorie count for the day could range from 1,285 to 1,735. It's going to depend on the food choices you make. When you stick to mostly low-fat foods, you'll come in closer to the low end of the range. You have a lot of flexibility built into this plan, however, and that allows you to eat, say, a baked apple with a drizzle of maple syrup and not worry so much about the calories in the syrup (as long as it's just a drizzle!). You can just count the apple as one of your fruit servings. This same flexibility makes it easier to eat at restaurants or other people's homes and not worry so much about every ingredient in the food. All you have to do is watch your portion sizes.

NutriTip
The amount of fat found naturally in food is taken into account in the open exchange plan. If you suspect there's a lot of extra fat in the food you're eating, you might want to check off one of your extra fat boxes.

Every time you eat, you simply check off the number of servings you've used up in each food group. For example, if you have a container of yogurt and a bran muffin for breakfast, you'll check one or two bread boxes (depending on the size of your muffin) and a milk/dairy box. If you grab a banana later in the morning, check off a fruit box. If you eat lunch out at a Chinese restaurant and you order beef with broccoli and white rice, check off the appropriate number of protein, vegetable, and bread boxes, depending on how much food you actually eat. At this point in the day, you should review your boxes and see what's left open.

That way you know what types of food you should choose to eat throughout the rest of the day to keep your diet balanced and within your calorie range.

Take It with You

Even though it's designed for a flexible schedule, there's no reason *not* to sit down to three regular meals a day while you're following the Open Exchange Plan. That is ideal, but when your schedule won't allow it, this check-box method lets you eat on the run or eat whatever is available to you. As some of the check boxes fill up during the day, the boxes that are still empty tell you the types of food choices you should try to make later in the day.

Some people like to make wallet-size copies of the 1,600 Calorie Open Exchange Checklist so it's easy to carry wherever they go. You may have your serving sizes down pat by now, but if not, refer to Chapter 13 for a review. If you're new at this, make a copy of the pyramid serving sizes and carry it along with your 1,600 Calorie Open Exchange Checklist.

Fair Exchanges

It's easy to figure out exchanges and serving sizes when you're eating individual foods that fit neatly into their respective food groups, such as a slice of bread, an apple, or a pork chop. However, combination foods such as casseroles, enchiladas, soups, and stews don't fit into single food groups. You'll come across many of these foods, and you'll just have to make an educated guess when you're figuring out how they fit into your eating plan. It's pretty much common sense when you break the food down into its parts. Often, when the food is prepared outside your home, it's wise to assume that there's some added fat in the dish. A bread exchange is often used to account for the calories in miscellaneous ingredients that don't fall into a group of their own or that don't have the nutritional value normally contributed by a food in that group. The following is a list of just a few combination foods and how they could fit into your eating plan:

Chili, meat or bean (1 cup): 2 breads, 1 meat, 1–2 fat

Chow mein (2 cups): 1 bread, 2 vegetable, 2 meat

Macaroni and cheese (1 cup): 2 bread, 1 milk/dairy, 1–2 fat

Pizza (1 slice): 2 breads, 1 milk/dairy, 1 fat

Pudding ($^1/_2$ cup): $^1/_2$ milk/dairy, 1 bread

Vegetable soup (canned; 1 cup): 1 bread

The Least You Need to Know

➤ There's more than one way to design an eating plan that will get you to a healthy weight.

➤ If you don't want to do any thinking or planning on your own, start with a straight menu plan that tells you exactly what to eat.

➤ Learn to modify your menu plan to include all the foods you enjoy eating.

➤ Even if you have an unusual schedule and can't stick to a routine menu plan, you can stick to your healthy eating plan by learning an exchange system based on serving sizes.

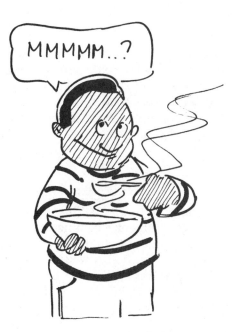

MMMMM..?

Chapter 22

The Low-Fat Kitchen

In This Chapter

➤ How to decipher the nutrition information on food labels

➤ Your supermarket is a health food store

➤ Stocking a healthy kitchen

Whenever I'm in line at the supermarket, I always sneak a look into other people's shopping carts to see what kind of foods they're buying. What I usually see is a mixed bag of fresh foods and convenience products—salad greens and low-fat dressings alongside frozen dinners and chocolate cookies. I see a lot of snacks and diet sodas. All in all, they're not much different from my own cart!

Eating to maintain a healthy weight starts with choosing the most nutritious foods at the market. Once you get those wholesome groceries home, you also have to make choices about how to prepare and cook them. No problem! Healthful food at its best is simple food. It doesn't require a lot of fuss and bother. This chapter will help you shop for the best food you can buy. You'll also learn how to stock your kitchen with the basic tools you need to get cooking.

Read All About It

It's not hard to pick out healthful foods at the supermarket now that all food packages wear Nutrition Facts labels. (These labels are now required by the Food and Drug Administration to ensure consumers get accurate, complete information.) Once you know how to read a Nutrition Facts label, you'll know how to make nutritious food choices. New food products arrive on the shelves all the time, and the hardest part about smart supermarket shopping is wading through the thousands of foods to choose from.

Just the Facts

To understand the information on the Nutrition Facts label found on packaged foods, you have to understand the Daily Values that the information is based on. That's easy.

NutriTip
Be sure to read the ingredient list found on all packaged foods. You might be surprised to find out exactly what your food is made of. Ingredients found in the largest amounts are listed first, and the rest are listed in descending order by weight.

Daily Values are the official government recommendations for the minimum or maximum amount of fat, saturated fat, cholesterol, sodium, carbohydrate, and fiber we should have in our diets. These recommendations are listed at the bottom of most Nutrition Facts labels, just as they are on the sample label shown on the following page.

If you eat more or less than 2,000 calories a day, the recommendations for these nutrients are somewhat higher or lower. The recommendations for a 2,500 calorie diet are also listed on the Nutrition Facts label. If you eat about 1,600 calories a day, your Daily Values are listed in Table 22.1.

Table 22.1   Daily Values Recommended for a 1,600-Calorie Diet

Nutrient	Amount (in grams)
Total Fat	Less than 53
Saturated Fat	Less than 18
Total Carbohydrate	240
Dietary Fiber	20*
Protein	46**

Minimum amount of fiber recommended for any calorie level below 2,000.
**Minimum amount of protein for any calorie level below 1,800.*

The recommended guidelines for cholesterol, sodium, most vitamins, and other minerals remain constant, regardless of your calorie level.

Food manufacturers are required to provide a % Daily Value column to show how a single serving of the food you're buying fits nutritionally into a daily 2,000 calorie diet. On the sample label, you can see that a 1-cup serving of this particular food contains 13 grams of fat per serving, or 20 percent of the Daily Value for fat.

Nutrition Facts

Serving Size 1 cup (228g)
Servings Per Container 2

Amount Per Serving

Calories 260 Calories from Fat 120

%Daily Value*

Total Fat 13g	20%
Saturated Fat 5g	25%
Cholesterol 30mg	10%
Sodium 660mg	28%
Total Carbohydrate 31g	10%
Dietary Fiber 0g	0%
Sugars 5g	
Protein 5g	

Vitamin A 4%	•	Vitamin C 2%	
Calcium 15%	•	Iron 4%	

*Percent Daily Values are based on a 2,000 calorie diet. Your daily values may be higher or lower depending on your calorie needs:

		Calories:	2,000	2,500
Total Fat	Less than		65g	80g
Sat Fat	Less than		20g	25g
Cholesterol	Less than		300mg	300mg
Sodium	Less than		2,400mg	2,400mg
Total Carbohydrate			300g	375g
Dietary Fiber			25g	30g

Calories per gram:

Fat 9 • Carbohydrate 4 • Protein 4

As you can see in the Daily Values listed near the bottom of the label, if you eat about 2,000 calories a day, your diet should contain less than 65 grams of fat. (Source: Food and Drug Administration, 1994)

Label Lingo

Now that the language on food labels is standardized, you can pick up a container of food and feel confident that what you see is what you get. Table 22.2 provides government definitions for some common food label terms you need to know when you're trying to lose weight.

Table 22.2   What It Means

Label Term	Meaning
Calorie free	Less than 5 calories per serving.
Reduced calorie	At least 25 percent fewer calories per serving than a similar food.
Low calorie	40 calories or less per serving.
Fat free or 100 percent fat free	Less than 0.5 gram per serving.
Reduced fat	At least 25 percent less fat per serving when compared with a similar food.
Saturated fat free	Less than 0.5 gram saturated fat.
Low saturated fat	1 gram or less saturated fat per serving and no more than 15 percent of calories from saturated fat.
Reduced saturated fat	At least 25 percent less saturated fat per serving when compared with a similar food.
Sugar free	Less than 0.5 grams sugar per serving.
Reduced sugar	At least 25 percent less sugar per serving when compared to a similar food.
No added sugars, Without added sugar	No amount of sugar or other ingredient that contains added sugars was added during processing; this claim can only be made if the product it resembles and substitutes for normally contains added sugar. (Remember that many foods contain natural sugars that are counted on the label.)

The Healthy Supermarket

I used to recommend sticking mostly to the outer aisles when shopping at the supermarket because that's where the healthiest foods could be found. It's still true that the freshest foods are found in the produce, meat, and dairy cases and those are usually found against the walls of the store. Now there's plenty of good, healthful food in *every* aisle. Let's take an aisle-by-aisle tour and find your best food bets in each.

Pick Your Produce

The best general advice anyone can give you for buying fresh fruits and vegetables is *buy in season*. For one thing, produce is cheaper when it's in season. For another, fruits and vegetables taste best when they're in season. The better your food tastes, the more you're going to want to eat it, right? Because many fruits and vegetables now come prewashed and precut, produce is practically a convenience food.

In fall and winter, seasonal vegetables include hard-skin squashes such as acorn, butternut, kabocha, delicata, sweet dumpling, and hubbard. Root vegetables such as turnips, rutabagas, and beets start to appear in the fall. Cabbage, Brussels sprouts, spinach, and fennel follow in mid-winter. Cold weather fruits include tangerines, kumquats, apples, and pears. Spring brings asparagus, artichokes, peas, and rhubarb. In summer, shop for corn, tomatoes, okra, peaches, plums, nectarines, melons, and berries.

NutriTip
Salad bars in supermarkets are an extension of the produce department and can come in handy when you're in a hurry and want to pick up fresh, ready-made side dishes for dinner.

Down Dairy Lane

If you're not savvy to the nutritional difference between low-fat and full-fat dairy products, just take a look at the labels. This example, using a cup of milk, demonstrates just how big the difference can be:

Milk, 1 cup	Calories	Fat (g)
Whole	149	8
2% low-fat	121	5
1% low-fat	100	3
Skim or nonfat	90	<1

The Meat Market

The meats that are most deceiving when it comes to fat are cold cuts and other processed meats such as hot dogs. That's because you can't see the fat when you look at a slice of bologna. Sometimes you can't even see it in a sausage, but you can be sure it's there!

You can't see all the fat in fresh meat either, only the obvious stuff that can be trimmed away. There's also fat in muscle, and the amount varies from cut to cut.

Lean cuts of beef

Eye of round	Top round
Top loin	Tenderloin
Sirloin	Chuck steaks or roasts
Cuts graded "select"	

Lean cuts of pork

Tenderloin	Top loin roast
Center loin chops	Loin rib chops
Shoulder blade chop	Lean ham

Lean cuts of lamb

Leg	Loin chop
Shoulder chop	Foreshank

Birdland

Most of the fat in a turkey or chicken is in and under the skin. That doesn't mean you have to buy a completely stripped bird just because you're watching your weight. Many people prefer to cook their turkey and chicken with the skin on to preserve moisture and flavor and then remove and discard the skin before they eat.

No Weigh!
Don't hesitate to buy chicken or turkey with the skin on. Fat from poultry skin doesn't travel into the meat during cooking, so it's okay to remove the skin just before you eat.

The darker meat in poultry has about three times as much fat and saturated fat as light meat, but in the context of an otherwise low-fat, balanced diet, it won't make a difference, especially if you're watching your portion sizes. Because domesticated duck and goose are darker-fleshed birds, their meat compares with the dark meat in other poultry.

If you're choosing ground turkey and chicken products to replace higher-fat ground meat, be sure to check the labels. There's no guarantee that a sausage or burger made with poultry is automatically low in fat.

Today's Catch

Most fish and shellfish are very low in fat. The leanest fish, with only 1 gram of fat or less in a 3-ounce serving, include cod, snapper, flounder, sole, crab, and scallops.

Even fattier fish, with four to seven or more grams of fat per serving, are relatively low-fat foods and should be included in your diet because the natural oils in these fish are thought to be "good" fats that may help lower blood cholesterol. These "fatty fish" include salmon, tuna, catfish, swordfish, trout, bluefish, and mackerel.

From the Freezer Case

You could build an entire meal from ingredients found in the freezer case, and it would be a pretty nutritious meal. Everything from appetizers to dessert can be found behind those glass doors or deep down in that chest. Some frozen foods are a little healthier than others, of course, and some are certainly better bets when you're watching your waistline. To name a few:

> **Guru's Corner**
> "Fish is the most healthful 'fast food' around. What's most essential is that fish be absolutely fresh. Get to know your fishmonger. The quality of fish is only as good as the person you buy it from. If it isn't always fresh, shop at another fish store."
>
> —David Ricketts, coauthor, *Simply Healthful Fish* (Houghton Mifflin/Chapters)

➤ **Unsweetened frozen fruit.** Thawed fruit makes its own juice, and you can use the mixture to top yogurt, waffles, or biscuits for breakfast or dessert.

➤ **Beans and greens.** Lima beans, black-eye beans, collards, kale, and mustard greens are available in frozen form. Although more and more fresh, nutritious greens are becoming available in markets all over the country, they're not always there when you need them.

➤ **Vegetable mixtures.** Instead of buying three or four different types of vegetables, you can get a lot of variety in a single bag. Stick with plain vegetable mixtures and season them yourself rather than take on the extra calories and possible fat that comes with a sauce.

➤ **Pasta.** Frozen plain ravioli and other filled pastas can be surprisingly low in fat. Check and compare labels.

➤ **Low-fat waffles.** Compare nutrition labels and choose the ones that have the most fiber.

➤ **Low-fat frozen dinners.** From a nutritional standpoint, I can't recommend thawing out a complete meal-in-a-box for dinner every night. But now that there are so many low-fat versions of these old-time favorite foods, it's okay to sneak one in once in a while in place of a real meal. (I certainly do!)

Cruisin' Down the Canned Food Aisle

If you asked me, I wouldn't recommend canned vegetables or fruit over fresh or frozen. Canning is a high-heat process that destroys some or all of the nutritional value of most foods. Let me also say this: Any canned food is better than no food at all. For anyone who's busy (and who isn't?), some canned foods make a whole lot more sense than fresh. The canned foods I most often recommend include

Tomatoes	Corn chowder
Tomato sauces	Corn kernels
Chicken broth	Beets
Vegetable broth	Tuna
Canned beans and lentils	Salmon
Split pea soup	Crab
Lentil soup	Sardines

Get Your Grain

One way to keep your food life exciting is to try new varieties of your favorite foods. If you eat a lot of pasta, switch shapes. Alongside the spaghetti and linguine, you'll find butterflies, wagon wheels, little ears, and angel hair. Look for whole wheat pasta that contains three times as much fiber as regular. Try pastas flavored with herbs, spinach, or tomato. They don't add more nutrients, just more fun. Sometimes that's just as important!

Guru's Corner
"Grains are easy to prepare but some take a while to cook. The good news is they freeze well and reheat well. They don't taste 'warmed over' like other leftovers. When you cook barley, cracked wheat, or other grains, make two or three times as much as you need and freeze what you don't use in ½ cup portions."

—Joanne Lamb Hayes, coauthor, *Grains: Seventy-Six Healthy Recipes for Barley, Corn, Rye, Wheat, and Other Grains* (Harmony Books, 1995)

While you're in the packaged food aisle, check out your rice choices. They're no longer limited to white or brown, instant or long-cooking. Most of the bigger markets now carry aromatic jasmine, jasmati, texmati, and basmati rices, alone and in blends. If you haven't tried them yet, you're in for a flavorful surprise. Many of the aromatic rices come in brown and white varieties. White cooks quicker, but keep in mind that brown rices have about three times as much fiber as white.

Don't forget about bulgur, buckwheat, couscous, spelt, barley, and other easy-to-prepare grains that are available in health food stores and large supermarkets. Many grains are now available in quick-cooking form and in preseasoned mixtures. If you buy whole grains plain and don't know what to do with them, start by substituting broth or orange juice for some or all of the water indicated in the basic cooking directions. From there, you can add herbs and sautéed seasoning vegetables such as onion, garlic, and mushrooms.

Taking Stock

Keep your cupboards stocked with a few basic foods so that when you don't have a meal plan and you're just too tired to think about it, you can still go home and know you'll find the makings of a meal. In addition to flour, sugar, baking soda, and other basics, a well stocked cupboard might contain

Sun-dried tomatoes and dried mushrooms

Tomato paste, tomato sauce, canned whole tomatoes

Canned meats and fish: chicken, tuna, salmon, crab

Shelf-stable or evaporated milk

Salsas, chutneys, and other low-fat condiments

Assorted pasta shapes

Assorted rices

Assorted grain mixes

Dried fruit

Canned beans and bean soups

Canned and powdered broths and bouillons

Canned fruits and vegetables

Nonstick vegetable oil cooking spray

Flavored vinegars

Fully Equipped

It doesn't take much to equip a kitchen for healthful cooking. As with healthful food, the simpler, the better. Beyond basic appliances, all you need are a few good pieces of equipment and utensils to match.

Magic in the Microwave

Microwave ovens are good weight-loss tools because food can be cooked with little or no added fat. In fact, the best foods to cook in a microwave oven are those you might normally steam, such as vegetables and seafood. Microwave ovens are also good for thawing

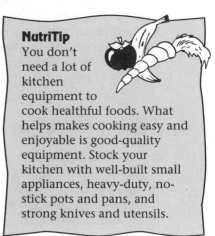

NutriTip
You don't need a lot of kitchen equipment to cook healthful foods. What helps makes cooking easy and enjoyable is good-quality equipment. Stock your kitchen with well-built small appliances, heavy-duty, no-stick pots and pans, and strong knives and utensils.

and reheating leftovers, and that might encourage you to cook large batches of grains, soups, stews, and other time-consuming foods to reheat for meals during the week. Here are some tips for using your microwave to prepare nutritious foods:

➤ Make sure the food you cook is cut into uniform-size pieces for even cooking. Larger, thicker pieces of food take longer to cook than smaller pieces.

➤ Foods at the outer edge of a dish will cook sooner than food located in the center of the dish. Faster-cooking foods should therefore be placed in the center. For example, to cook broccoli spears in a pie plate, you arrange the broccoli so the thicker stems face the outer edge of the dish and the flowerets face the center. If you're cooking carrots and zucchini together, arrange the carrots in a ring around the outer edge and the zucchini in the center of the dish.

➤ In most cases, you should cover food with a lid or with microwave-safe plastic wrap to hold in moisture and heat and ensure more even cooking.

➤ When food is removed from a microwave oven, it continues to cook. Very dense dishes, such as casseroles, may continue cooking for up to 15 or 20 minutes. Recipes adapted for microwave cooking usually take this time factor into consideration.

➤ Always uncover a microwave dish carefully and starting with the side that points away from you to avoid steam burns.

All Steamed Up

Steamers are used throughout the world to cook healthful foods of all kinds, especially vegetables and seafood. Trapped steam cooks the food by moist heat so there's no need for added fat. You're probably familiar with the inexpensive collapsible metal steamer basket that can be inserted into a saucepan. Those are the easiest to find, but I find them to be the clumsiest to use for anything that can't be removed from the pan easily using tongs. If you're serious about steaming, you might be better off with a Chinese stackable bamboo steamer that can cook a couple of levels of food at once. It's much easier to remove the food from a bamboo steamer once it's been cooked. Bamboo steamers are available at most specialty cookware shops. Electric rice cookers also double as steamers, as do the perforated draining baskets that come with pasta pots. If you own either of these pieces of equipment, a separate steamer might not be necessary.

One Good Knife (or Two)

If you could have only one good knife, pick an eight- to ten-inch chef's knife to use for chopping and slicing. If you can have two, pick a chef's knife and a paring knife for peeling and trimming. You get what you pay for, and you'll probably pay at least $50 for the chef's knife and $20 for the paring knife. The best quality knives are usually made from high-carbon non-staining steel. The blade should extend into the full length of the handle. Make sure the knife feels comfortable in your hand before you buy it. If you've never owned a good quality knife, you'll notice the difference with your very first cut.

Just Basics

There's so much equipment and so many tools you could have in your kitchen, but unless you're a hopeless "gadgeteer," you really need only a few basics. If you're just starting out, start with the items on this list:

➤ Food processor or blender

➤ Citrus juicer (reamer)

➤ Dry measuring cups

➤ Liquid measuring cups

➤ Measuring spoons

➤ No-stick cookware:

Large, medium, and small skillet

Large, medium, and small saucepan

Very large saucepan or Dutch oven

Lids

➤ No-stick bakeware:

Two round cakes pans

One square cake pan

One 9-inch pie plate

Two cookie sheets

One 12-cup muffin pan

➤ No-stick utensils

➤ Rubber spatulas

➤ Wooden spoons

➤ Slotted spoon

➤ Wire mesh sieve

Guru's Corner

"A good knife is worth the investment because it will last a lifetime if you take care of it. Don't stick it in the dishwasher or throw it in a drawer with other cutlery. Clean your knife by hand and store it in a knife block, on a wall-mounted magnetic knife holder, or in its own sheath."

—Michael Krondl, instructor, New School Culinary Center, New York

The Least You Need to Know

➤ The Nutrition Facts label found on all packaged foods is a valuable tool for choosing the most nutritious foods in the supermarket.

➤ Buy fresh fruits and vegetables during their peak seasons for the best flavor and the best prices.

➤ If you choose carefully and read labels, you'll find plenty of canned and frozen foods in the supermarket that are low in fat and high in good nutrition.

➤ All you need to stock a kitchen for healthy cooking are a few basic pieces of good-quality equipment.

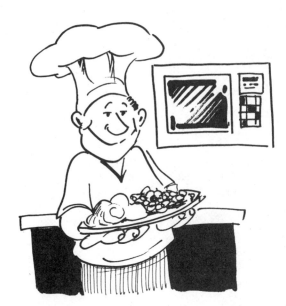

Chapter 23

Let's Cook!

In This Chapter

➤ One simple soup with endless variations

➤ A creamy low-fat dressing for all your salad needs

➤ Very simple main dishes

➤ Side dish selections

➤ What's for dessert?

➤ Low-fat substitutes for everyday ingredients

For everyday low-fat cooking, all you need are a few good, basic recipes to work from. This chapter provides easy answers to that age-old question of what to have for supper. Nothing fancy. Nothing you can't handle at the end of a busy day.

Soup's On!

Here's how you can make a variety of nutritious soups from a single recipe.

Creamy Any-Vegetable Soup

Makes four servings.

Per serving: 169 calories, 4 grams fat

½ bread servings, 1 vegetable serving

Variations: This recipe is the base for all kinds of low-fat, creamy vegetable soup mixtures. Instead of carrots, you could use broccoli, cauliflower, winter squash, beets, or roasted peppers. Season with your favorite herbs and spices.

> 2 teaspoons vegetable oil
>
> 1 onion, finely chopped
>
> ¾ pound all-purpose potatoes, peeled and diced
>
> ½ pound carrots, peeled and cut up
>
> 1 can (13¾ ounces) reduced-sodium chicken broth
>
> 1 cup skim milk
>
> ⅛ teaspoon nutmeg
>
> Salt and pepper to taste

Heat the oil in a large saucepan over medium heat. Add onion; cook for five minutes or until tender. Add the potatoes, carrots, and chicken broth. Heat to boiling. Reduce heat to medium-low; partially cover and simmer ten minutes or until the potatoes are tender.

Use a slotted spoon to transfer half the vegetables to a blender or food processor. Add a little broth and process until smooth. Return the mixture to the saucepan. (If you prefer a completely smooth soup, puree all the vegetables.) Stir in the milk and nutmeg. Taste and add salt and pepper, if necessary. Heat through and serve.

Salad Fixin's

All you need to dress up a bowl of leafy salad greens is a drizzle of this fresh, creamy vinaigrette.

Yogurt Vinaigrette

Makes six servings (¼ cup each).

Per serving: 33 calories, 1 gram fat

¼ milk/dairy serving

Variations: There are so many ways to vary this vinaigrette. Use flavored vinegars instead of wine vinegar or lime juice instead of lemon juice. Add herbs such as dill or tarragon, or try a pinch of curry powder, chili powder, or Cajun or Italian seasoning. You can even turn this into a dressing for a savory fruit salad such as spinach with pears. To do so, leave out the garlic and pepper and add a drizzle of honey and some poppy seeds.

1 container (8 ounces) low-fat plain yogurt

¼ cup buttermilk or 2 tablespoons low-fat milk

2 tablespoons white wine vinegar

1 tablespoon lemon juice

1 teaspoon Dijon mustard

1 clove garlic, pressed or finely chopped

⅛ teaspoon ground black pepper

Combine all the ingredients in a covered jar and shake gently to combine. (You can also whisk ingredients together in a small bowl.) Cover and refrigerate for up to one week.

The Main Course

Because they lend themselves to so many simple variations, the following meals just might be the only four main-dish recipes you'll ever need.

Chicken Cutlets with Lemon and Basil

Makes four servings.

Per serving: 139 calories, 2 grams fat

1 meat serving

Variations: You can substitute thinly sliced chicken, pork, or veal cutlets for the turkey in this recipe. If you're using pork or veal, you can also substitute equal amounts of sage or thyme for the basil.

1 tablespoon all-purpose flour

⅛ teaspoon salt

1 pound thin chicken cutlets

⅛ teaspoon ground pepper

½ cup reduced-sodium chicken broth

1 tablespoon lemon juice

¼ cup finely chopped fresh basil or 1 teaspoon dried basil

Combine flour and salt in a plastic food bag. Add cutlets and toss to coat.

Lightly coat a large nonstick skillet with nonstick cooking spray. Place the skillet over medium-high heat. Add the cutlets and cook two minutes or until golden on underside. Turn cutlets over, sprinkle with pepper, and cook two minutes longer. Add chicken broth and lemon juice. Sprinkle with basil. Reduce heat to medium; simmer one minute longer or until cutlets are just cooked through.

Transfer the cutlets to dinner plate, spoon pan liquid over, and serve.

Garlic and Herb Meat Rub

Makes four servings.

Per serving: 178 calories, 7 grams fat

1 meat serving

Variations: You can substitute lamb steaks or pork chops for the beef and use oregano or thyme instead of the rosemary. Add a tablespoon of lemon juice to the rub if you use lamb or pork.

> 2 large cloves garlic, pressed
>
> 1 tablespoon dried rosemary, crumbled
>
> ¼ teaspoon salt
>
> 1 pound sirloin steak

Preheat the broiler. Combine the garlic, rosemary, and salt in a small bowl. Rub the mixture into both sides of the steak. Arrange the steak on a broiler pan.

Broil steak four inches from heat until cooked through, about four to six minutes on each side for medium.

Orange-Soy Glazed Cod Steaks

Makes four servings.

Per serving: 136 calories, 1 gram fat

1 meat serving

Variations: You can substitute any fish steak, such as halibut, swordfish, shark, or salmon, for the cod steaks.

> ¼ cup orange juice
>
> 2 tablespoons reduced-sodium soy sauce
>
> 2 tablespoons honey

1 clove garlic, pressed

1 pound cod steaks or thick fillets

Combine the juice, soy sauce, honey, and garlic in a medium-size bowl. Add cod steaks and turn to coat. Marinate in the refrigerator for at least 30 minutes or up to 4 hours.

Preheat the broiler. Line the broiler pan with aluminum foil.

Broil the fish four inches from the heat until browned on top and opaque all the way through, about four to six minutes.

Janine D'Amato's Vegetarian BBQ-on-a-Bun

Makes four servings.

Per serving: 335 calories, 4 grams fat

2 bread servings, 1-ounce meat alternative, 1 vegetable serving

Variations: You can substitute white beans, pinto beans, black beans, or lentils for the kidney beans in this recipe and add any vegetables you like. You can use 2 cups rice or 2 cups corn instead of 1 cup of each. This mixture is also delicious over corn bread.

1 teaspoon vegetable oil

1 onion, finely chopped

1 sweet red pepper, finely chopped

1 can (19 ounces) kidney beans (2 cups), drained and lightly rinsed

1 cup cooked rice

1 cup corn kernels

½ cup Kansas City-style or smoky barbecue sauce

2 hamburger buns, split

Heat the oil in a large nonstick skillet over medium heat. Add onion and pepper; sauté five minutes or until tender. Stir in beans, rice, corn, and barbecue sauce. Cook until hot and bubbly, about five minutes.

Place a bun half on each plate. Spoon BBQ mixture over buns and serve.

On the Side

What do you have to do to make vegetables taste good? Not much! Here are some simple ideas.

Steamed Vegetables with Herbs

Steam cut-up vegetables for five to ten minutes or until tender-crisp. The easiest way to jazz up steamed vegetables is to enhance their flavor with fresh or dried herbs. Use the following list of herbs as a guide to seasoning your favorite vegetables. Although most herbs go well with most any vegetable, some are natural partners.

➤ Basil with tomatoes, eggplant, zucchini, and yellow summer squash

➤ Dill with beets, carrots, and cucumbers

➤ Oregano with tomatoes, cabbage, and salad greens

➤ Parsley with potatoes, grains, and tomatoes

➤ Rosemary with peas, green beans, spinach, zucchini, and yellow squash

➤ Sage with onions, mushrooms, and salad greens

➤ Tarragon with mushrooms, carrots, and salad greens

➤ Thyme with mushrooms, okra, zucchini, yellow squash, and salad greens

Creamy Twice-Baked Potatoes

Makes four servings.

Per serving: 292 calories, 3 grams fat

2 bread servings, 1 milk/dairy serving

Variations: You can use chives, vidalia, or sweet red onions in place of the green onions. You can also add an herb, such as basil or dill, to the potato mixture.

4 medium-size baking potatoes (about 1¾ pounds)

½ cup shredded reduced-fat Monterey Jack, Swiss, Mozzarella, or Cheddar cheese

¾ cup nonfat plain yogurt

¼ cup finely chopped green onion

⅛ teaspoon salt

⅛ teaspoon pepper

Preheat the oven to 400 degrees. Bake the potatoes for one hour or until tender. Remove potatoes from oven and increase temperature to 450 degrees.

Cut a thin slice from the top of each potato and scoop out the flesh into a small bowl, leaving the potato shells intact. Add cheese, yogurt, onion, salt, and pepper to bowl. Stir and mash mixture together. Carefully stuff the mixture back into the potato shells. Place potatoes on a baking sheet, bake for 15 minutes longer, and serve.

Sweet Stuff

These quick, fruity desserts also make great afternoon snacks.

Quickie "Baked" Apple

Makes one serving.

Per serving: 165 calories, 1 gram fat

1 bread serving, 1 fruit serving

Variation: You can substitute low-fat granola or muesli for the Grape Nuts and use honey, molasses, or brown sugar in place of maple syrup.

> 1 medium-size apple
>
> 2 tablespoons Grape Nuts cereal
>
> 2 teaspoons maple syrup

Peel the apple halfway down from the top and cut out the core. Stuff the apple with the cereal and syrup. Place in a microwave-safe bowl and cover loosely with plastic wrap. Microwave on high for 1 to 2 minutes or until softened. Uncover and let stand for 1 minute before serving.

Pears with Strawberry Cream

Makes two servings.

Per serving: 185 calories, 2 grams fat

1 milk/dairy serving, 1 fruit serving

> 1 firm-ripe pear
>
> 1 cup fresh or dry-pack frozen strawberries, thawed
>
> 1 cup low-fat (1 percent) cottage cheese
>
> 1 tablespoon honey or sugar

Cut the pear in half, scoop out the core, and cut into thin slices. Place the slices in a microwave-safe dish. Cover and microwave on high power for 30 seconds.

Set one strawberry aside. Combine the remaining strawberries, cheese, and honey in the container of a food processor or blender. Process one minute or until very smooth, scraping down side of container as necessary.

Divide strawberry-cheese mixture among dessert cups. Add pear slices. Halve remaining strawberry and use as a garnish.

Good Substitutes

Beyond the obvious substitutes for certain high-fat foods, such as replacing regular sour cream with a reduced-fat or fat-free version in recipes, there are low-fat substitutes you can quickly whip up in your own kitchen. They not only taste better than many of the modified products on the market, but they are also more nutritious. Table 23.1 lists great substitutions that you can use to reduce the fat content in your favorite recipes.

Table 23.1 Low-Fat Substitutes

Instead of	Try
Sour cream	Pureed cottage cheese* or low-fat plain yogurt or a half-and-half combination of pureed cottage cheese and yogurt as a cold topping or in baked goods such as cakes and muffins.
Creamy salad dressings	Plain yogurt or pureed cottage cheese, or a combination, flavored with lemon juice or flavored vinegars, mustard, herbs, or small amounts of full-flavored soft cheese such as blue cheese or dry seasoning mixes.
Cream cheese	Pureed "light" ricotta cheese mixed together with an equal amount of fat-free cream cheese.
Butter or margarine	Applesauce, prune butter**, mashed ripe banana in baking, or other commercial or homemade fruit-based puree. You can replace all but a tablespoon or two of the fat indicated in most recipes for cakes, brownies, muffins, and other baked goods with fruit purees. Remember, however, that the texture of the final product will be different from the original.

To make pureed cottage cheese or ricotta cheese, simply place cheese in the container of a blender or food processor and process until very smooth, about one minute.

**To make prune puree, combine 1 cup of pitted prunes with 1 cup of water in a medium-size saucepan; simmer until prunes are tender, about 5 minutes. Place the mixture in a food processor or blender. Add another cup of water and process until very smooth, about one minute. (You'll have about 1½ cups of puree you can store in the refrigerator for at least a week.)*

The Least You Need to Know

➤ It's not always what you eat that helps you gain weight, but how you prepare it. The recipes in this chapter make the most of healthful cooking techniques and ingredients, and you can easily adapt them to suit your own taste.

➤ You can start cutting back on fat right now by substituting lower fat ingredients wherever you can in your favorite recipes.

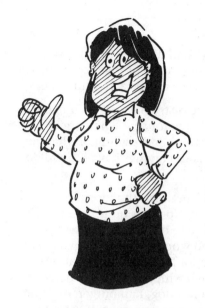

Chapter 24

No Problem!

In This Chapter

➤ What to do about cravings

➤ Advice for snackers

➤ How to have your dessert and eat it too

➤ Figuring in your favorite fast foods

➤ How to cope with traveling, partying, and other situations that can threaten a healthy eating plan

You're not immune to the trappings of real life while you're trying to lose or maintain weight. You'll still get cravings for French fries, you'll want to eat sweet desserts, or you won't be able to kick your peanut butter snack habit. All of these situations are manageable, however, so don't sweat it.

This chapter gives you real solutions for those very real food challenges you face from day to day.

Cravings

When you get a craving, it's probably not for a crisp green salad drizzled with low-fat dressing. More likely, your cravings are for foods that are high in fat or sugar or both. You probably crave something such as a triple-fudge brownie bar or maybe a 16-ounce steak.

Hormones, self-indulgence, emotional upsets, and brain chemistry have all been blamed for food cravings, but scientists who study cravings don't know for sure where these irresistible urges originate. They do agree that there's something more going on than just a simple longing for a favorite food. One thing's for sure: Your cravings have little to do with actual hunger.

NutriTip
Allow yourself to eat the foods you crave in reasonable amounts on a regular basis, rather than avoid them altogether. If you deprive yourself completely of foods you enjoy, you're more likely to overeat when you finally give in to a craving.

There seems to be a difference between the foods women crave and the foods men crave. No one's quite sure what this is about, but it might have to do with the different hormones that drive men and women's behavior. Generally, a woman is more likely to go for fat-sugar combinations such as chocolate or sweetened whipped cream, whereas a man is more likely to crave a hot dog, hamburger, or some other fat-protein combo. Whatever you crave, if you can satisfy your urges with small indulgences here and there, you're less likely to find yourself eating an entire container of whipped topping or a bag of potato chips the size of a pillowcase.

Snack-Size Solutions

Are you a sneaky snacker? Always popping something into your mouth when no one's looking and then feeling guilty? Get over it! Most people love to snack and it's only a problem if your snack habit gets out of control and starts contributing to your weight gain. If that's the case, there are simple solutions.

Solution #1

Allow yourself to snack but have just one rule: All snacks must be from one of the five pyramid food groups. (The fats and sweets group at the tip of the pyramid doesn't count here!) That gives you a wide range of allowable snack foods, including

Cereals

Crackers

Toasts

Waffles

Fresh fruits

Frozen fruits

Canned fruits

Raw vegetables

Reduced-fat cheeses (in small amounts!)

Reduced-sodium pickles

Yogurts

Solution #2

Clear the house of junk foods. The rationale here is if you can't see it, you won't be tempted to eat it. Of course, that won't stop you from going out and buying whatever food you feel like eating, but the extra effort might make you think twice. Instead, keep the fridge packed with cut-up fruits and vegetables, ready-to-eat yogurt dips, and other low-fat snack foods.

Solution #3

Schedule snacks into your daily routine. Plan your snacks as mini meals. To do that, be sure you're getting some carbohydrate, protein, and a little fat at every snack, just as you do at every meal. If, for example, you normally eat a bag of tortilla chips every afternoon, create a plan around that choice. Instead of just chips, schedule an afternoon snack that includes a reasonable number of low-fat chips (10 or 12), some fresh salsa, and maybe a small piece of cheese. Now you're eating a small, fairly well-rounded meal that includes foods from three different food groups. Snack this way, and you're likely to stay full longer and be less tempted to snack again before your regular meal.

Solution #4

Be creative. Just because your snacks are essentially good for you, that doesn't mean they have to be dull. The following are few of my favorite instant snack combos:

➤ Toasted whole-grain waffle topped with sliced peaches and vanilla-maple yogurt (and maybe a few walnuts).

➤ Multi-grain saltine crackers topped with sliced cherry tomatoes and shredded, reduced-fat mozzarella cheese. (Melt in toaster oven or microwave.)

➤ Toasted cinnamon-raisin bagel half topped with reduced-fat ricotta cheese and sliced strawberries.

➤ Toasted oat-bran English muffin half spread with apple butter and topped with apple slices and shredded cheddar or crumbled blue cheese. (Melt in toaster oven or microwave.)

Sweet Surrender

Supermarket shelves are loaded down with fat-free cookies, cakes, and pastries, but unfortunately, these desserts aren't much healthier than their fat-laden sisters and brothers. That's because when the fat comes out, something else has to go in to take its place, and that something is usually sugar. Fat-free desserts end up with almost as many calories as those that still

No Weigh!
Don't fall into the fat-free trap. Desserts that are fat-free are usually high in sugar and often contain just as many calories as the original full-fat version. Check the label to see if a low-fat food is high in calories.

contain fat. Because they're labeled "fat-free," however, you can be fooled into thinking these products won't cause weight gain. Wrong!

Fruity Treats

You can have dessert every day and eat it without feeling guilty and without worrying that it will ruin your healthy eating plan. Here's how. When you have a choice, pick a dessert that satisfies something more than your sweet tooth (and the fat tooth behind it). Choose a dessert that also satisfies a nutritional need because it supplies some protein, vitamins, minerals, or fiber. The obvious choice is fresh fruit, but sometimes a plain old orange at the end of a meal just doesn't cut it. Look for dessert recipes that use fresh fruit in creative, satisfying ways by baking, sautéing, or grilling the fruit with just a little fat or sugar. Here are some ideas for fruit desserts that can satisfy your need for sweet stuff but still pack some nutritional punch:

NutriTip
Fruit becomes a more satisfying dessert when you bake it, poach it, grill it, or cook it in the microwave oven and sweeten it just slightly with a little sugar or honey. Make it a goal to find fun new ways to prepare fruit desserts.

Poached pears

Baked apple

Grilled pineapple

Sautéed banana slices

Fruit crumble

Fruit compote

Stewed fruit

Cheese and fresh fruit platter

Healthier Baking

When you're making dessert, use these tips to make it more healthful:

➤ Choose dessert recipes that use fruit or vegetables, such as a carrot cake or pumpkin pie. If your recipes haven't been developed to be low in fat, learn to modify them with fruit-based fat substitutes (see "Good Substitutes" in Chapter 23, "Let's Cook!").

➤ Look for recipes that call for vegetable oil rather than butter or margarine. (You can still replace some of that fat with fruit-based substitutes.)

➤ Substitute whole wheat flour for half of the white flour called for in the recipe.

➤ Substitute two egg whites for each whole egg indicated in the recipe. You can do this with some or all of the eggs. If the recipe calls for two eggs, you use one whole egg plus two whites or you can use four egg whites.

➤ Cut down just a little on the total amount of sugar. If the recipe calls for 1 cup, try making it with ¾ cup.

Special Situations

The way you eat has to fit in with your normal, everyday life. When you travel, eat out at restaurants, celebrate special occasions, or pick up a quick meal at a fast food chain, don't worry about whether you can stick to your healthy eating plan. Of course you can!

Travel

Depending on where you're going and your mode of travel, you might want to brown bag it rather than risk having nothing to eat but "road food." Your best bet is to plan ahead. If you're taking a trip in the car, you can bring an insulated chest to hold whatever foods you want. Even if you're headed out on a bus or a train, you can pack a small selection of convenience foods that don't require refrigeration—anything that will keep you away from the club car or the vending machines at bus stops. Here are some ideas:

Individual boxes of cold cereal

Packets of instant hot cereal

Individual containers of applesauce and puddings

Small "pop" cans of fruit

Shelf-stable low-fat milk

Small plastic bottles of water

My friend Joyce packs a knife, fork, and spoon in her carry-bag whenever she goes to Paris. That way she's always prepared to have her favorite French picnic meal: crusty bread, a small hunk of cheese, and a piece of fresh fruit. Even if you're not headed for Europe, it might pay to pack some utensils when you travel. That way, you won't be limited to restaurant or hotel food. You can pick up a healthy meal or snack anywhere. You not only stand the chance of saving calories, but you'll probably save money, too.

Advice from Losers

"Even though I work with food, I go to a lot of food parties, and I travel a great deal on food trips, I lost 80 pounds in a year and a half and I can't believe how easy it actually was. After years of reading diet books and trying to figure out how to eat in the same way as a 'normal' person, I realized there is no norm. There's no one way to eat except the way you decide is best for yourself. Basically I just had to trust myself. I stopped looking for gimmicks, balanced my diet, and learned how to make appropriate choices. I can eat whatever I want now because I eat more consciously."

—Mitchell D.

Eating Out

If you really want to be careful about how you eat out, start by choosing a restaurant that offers a selection of "light" or "heart-healthy" dishes. Choose a restaurant that features a naturally low-fat cuisine, such as a Japanese or seafood restaurant. When in doubt, ask how the dish you want to order is prepared. Ask what's in it and how it's cooked. If you think the dish could be prepared differently, ask whether the chef is willing to use a different cooking method.

You might want to "bank" some calories and eat lighter meals during the day when you know you're going out to eat that night. You could also put some extra time into your workout. Whatever you do, don't starve yourself in anticipation of a special meal. Going without food will only lead to overeating when you finally have a meal. Eating a small snack about half an hour before you go out to eat can help cut your appetite so you have more control over the amount of food you eat at your meal. Here are some other tips for healthier restaurant eating:

➤ Stay away from all-you-can-eat buffets unless you feel confident that most of your selections are low in fat.

➤ If it doesn't come automatically, ask for water as soon as you sit down.

➤ Start your meal with a clear (not creamy) soup.

➤ Always order a large green salad to have before your meal.

➤ Order salad dressings, sauces, gravies, butter, and sour cream on the side.

➤ When eating out with someone else, order an appetizer each and split an entree.

➤ Search the menu for dishes that are poached, steamed, boiled, broiled, or grilled.

➤ Ask the waiter to take the butter dish away from the table.

➤ If you tend to load up on bread before your meal, ask the waiter to take the basket away until the entrees are served.

➤ Share dessert. Order whatever you want, but don't have it all to yourself.

➤ Have a flavored coffee for dessert.

Fast Food

In an ideal weight-loss world, there is always time to shop for fresh food and cook all our meals from scratch so that we can have better control over what we eat. Ha! Not in this lifetime. Nowadays we have no choice but to rely on convenience foods for so many of our meals. For many of us, convenience means eating out at fast-food restaurants or picking up a sandwich at the deli. Believe it or not, you can eat hamburgers, hot dogs, tacos, pizza, or any favorite fast food when you're trying to lose or maintain weight. You can't get away with eating a *lot* of these foods, but if you don't overdo it and you're willing to do a little planning, you don't have to give them up completely. Here are some suggestions for fitting in fast foods:

➤ Have a plan. If you plan your menus for the day, you can always figure out a way to include a hamburger or taco lunch. Have a lean, high-fiber breakfast and plan a light dinner of say, broiled fish and vegetables, for later the same day.

➤ Order only regular-size portions. Skip deluxe, large, and super sizes.

➤ Order just one—one hamburger, one taco, one slice of pizza.

➤ Don't go overboard. Instead of a hamburger, fries, and a thick shake, choose one higher-fat item and surround it with lower-calorie and lower-fat foods such as soups and salads.

➤ Try to skip condiments other than ketchup and mustard, or ask for low-fat mayonnaise, tartar sauce, or salad dressing.

Celebrate!

Holidays, birthdays, promotions, anniversaries—there's always something to celebrate, and celebrations always involve food. If the party's at your house, you have a lot more control over the food. You can also plan a party that focuses more on an activity than on food. Parties for kids almost always include some form of entertainment besides eating, so why not do the same at parties for adults? Have an origami party, invite a guest speaker or a dance instructor, or set up a volleyball net. However, you can't assume there will be low-fat foods or entertaining diversions at other people's parties. When in doubt, here's what you can do:

➤ Eat something before you go to the party.

➤ Contribute to a platter of low-fat food to the party.

➤ Don't plant yourself in front of the paté platter.

➤ Keep a glass of water in your hand at all times.

➤ Get involved in conversations so you're talking instead of eating.

The Least You Need to Know

➤ It's better to occasionally indulge in the foods you crave than to deprive yourself and overeat when you finally give in.

➤ If you treat snacks like little meals, they won't get in the way of a healthy eating plan.

➤ You don't ever have to skip dessert, even when you're trying to lose weight. You just have to make sensible choices.

➤ The best way to cope with parties, traveling, eating out, and other challenges to healthy eating is to plan ahead.

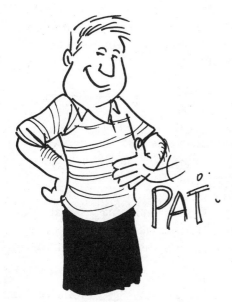

PAT.

Chapter 25

Keep Up the Good Work!

In This Chapter

➤ What to do when you reach a weight plateau

➤ Maintaining your weight

➤ Passing your fitness lessons on to your children

I can't tell you how many people have said to me, "I can lose the weight, but I can't keep it off." That's the same as saying a weight-loss diet "worked" even though you put the pounds back on and then some. Maintaining weight loss *is* impossible if you go on and off weight-loss diets or if you give up before you get to your goal. But if you've read this far, you already know that.

If you've hit a weight plateau or you've reached your healthy weight, this chapter is for you. This is where you'll learn what it takes to maintain the weight you've worked so hard to achieve. Here's a clue: Not much is new!

When You Reach a Plateau

It happens to everyone who's trying to lose weight. There you are, moving right along and doing everything you're supposed to do, when suddenly you hit a weight plateau. Nothing budges. It seems as though no matter what you do, you can't lose an ounce. A plateau can last for a couple of weeks or, sorry to say, it can last for months. Plateaus are different for everyone. Whatever you do, don't give up! Muster up all your patience and all your faith and hang in there. Every plateau eventually breaks.

Advice from Losers

"I've always been overweight. It's on my mother's side of the family. I've tried to lose weight half a dozen times and I can always lose 40 pounds, but then I plateau and don't see any results for a long time. That's when I used to give up. When I look back at my old diaries, I see the same pattern over and over again. I told myself this last time that I would stick with my plan no matter what. I've just broken through a plateau that lasted five months. I tried many things. The most recent was working out with weights for the first time. I think that helped the most."

—Pat D.

Stay Calm

Do a self-check. Are you sticking to your diet plan? Are you exercising as much as ever? Be sure none of your "old ways" has crept back before you declare yourself at a plateau.

You can't worry away a plateau. Instead, take positive measures to keep your motivation high when you're not losing. Whatever you do, don't weigh yourself every day. Getting on a scale can be too discouraging when the numbers temporarily get stuck. If you belong to a weight-loss group, try to attend more meetings and ask if plateaus can be a topic for discussion. It helps to get reassurance from those who've been there. Don't let negative thoughts take over. If necessary, go back to Chapter 4, "Heavy Thoughts," and Chapter 20, "Thinking Fit," for a review on positive self-talk and affirmations. Appendix B, "Your Best Resources," lists other publications and organizations that can help you deal with the emotional aspects of losing weight. Check them out.

Plateau Busters

You can't predict how long your plateau will last, and often there's not much you can do about it except keep up the good work you're already doing and wait it out. At the same time, you can shift the status quo by making small, temporary changes in the way you eat or the way you exercise. Here are some ideas:

➤ Make sure you're drinking at least eight to ten 8-ounce cups of water a day.

➤ Change your diet. If you're eating the same foods at the same time every day, figure out a way to break the pattern for just a week. For example, if you normally eat cereal every day for breakfast, try having yogurt, cottage cheese, or eggs and lean ham instead. Just make a small, single change without drastically altering the basic eating plan that's been working for you so far.

➤ Change your exercise. If you have an exercise routine, try breaking it. If you've been running for 30 minutes on a treadmill at your gym, try putting in 10 of those minutes on a rowing machine or stair climber. If you haven't been pushing yourself lately, try increasing the amount of time you spend exercising each day, even if it's only by five minutes.

No Weigh!
Don't get discouraged and certainly don't give up when you hit a weight-loss plateau. Try to shift your body's balance by changing your diet slightly or exercising differently. It might take longer than you like, but you *will* start to lose weight again.

Weight Maintenance

This is your life. It's no longer about going on quick-fix diets or frantically trying to figure out how to lose ten pounds before your sister's (or your own) wedding. When you made a decision to get to a healthy weight, you decided to make changes in your life. You chose to live a healthier, more active lifestyle than the one you were living before. Weight maintenance means an ongoing commitment to that new lifestyle. There are two stages of weight loss when you need to think about maintenance:

NutriTip
To maintain your healthy weight, you have to stay committed to the lifestyle choices that helped you lose the weight in the first place. Keep exercising and eating well, and you'll stay fit.

➤ When you hit a plateau
➤ When you reach your healthy weight goal

What You Know

If you've followed along in this book and used it to get to your healthy weight, there's little you don't know about keeping your mind and body fit. From here on in, it's all reinforcement. But wait! That doesn't mean doing the same old thing over and over again for the rest of your life. It means that these basic principles you learned about *getting* fit also apply to *staying* fit:

➤ Eat nutritionally balanced meals.
➤ Get some type of regular exercise.
➤ Keep a positive outlook.
➤ Don't ever give up.

I know there was a time when you would have read these rules, raised your eyebrows, and thought "Sure, that's easy for you to say." When you started on your journey to lose weight, there was nothing easy about following any of these rules. That's because you had to discover for yourself what each one meant and what it takes for you to be able to apply these principles to your own life. Now you know.

Stick to It

You already have a solid plan for getting to a healthy weight, and that's the plan you're going to use to maintain it. In other words, whatever you've been doing is working, so stick to it. The big difference between losing and maintaining is that instead of learning how to have a healthier lifestyle, you can start living it. But you're still practicing. Don't be tempted to give up any of the tools that helped you lose weight—not yet. If you belong to a weight-loss group or are involved in any type of counseling that's helped you lose the weight, don't drop out.

More Change

Change is a recurring theme throughout this book because it's the first thing you had to do to lose weight. You had to change something about the way you eat, exercise, and think. Remember this: You're still changing, and you're still adjusting to the many changes you've already made. It's important to stay flexible. You're at your healthy weight, and staying there will take the same amount of patience and openness to change that it took to get there. Nothing is ending or beginning. You're simply moving from one stage of weight control to another.

Go Back

No matter how committed you are to living a healthier lifestyle, there's always a chance you'll meet a situation that will threaten your resolve to stay fit—especially if overeating is something you used to do to deal with stress and emotions. Get it before it gets you. Gather all your resources and, if need be, go back to the beginning. I hope you've filled in the workbook pages of this book and kept food diaries and journals along the way. Pick them up and read them again for motivation. Your diaries and scribblings serve as a reminder of where you once were in your struggle against weight loss and how hard you had to work to get where you are now. Reading those notes again might give you more determination when your best intentions aren't enough.

Move Forward

Always be on the lookout for new resources to help you maintain a healthier lifestyle and keep fitness fun. Buy new cookbooks, keep up with new styles of exercise, try out new foods, and read new fitness magazines. Keep setting new goals for your life and your health. Your lifestyle is a work in progress and that means constantly updating yourself, expanding your interests, and setting new goals so you're always moving forward.

Pass It Down!

Now that you've whipped yourself into shape, what about the rest of your family? If you read the "Advice from Losers" sidebars throughout this book, you probably noticed that many of these contributors come from overweight families and have been heavy most of their lives. Some of them told me they were passing the same bad habits on to their own children. Others were able to turn around and change the way their parents approach fitness. Now that you know what you know about thinking and acting fit, you might be able to do the same with your family.

> **NutriTip**
> After the age of two, it's a good idea to start introducing your child to healthy eating habits and using the food guide pyramid as a teaching tool.

If you're a parent, you can help your children stay fit by setting them on the right nutritional and exercise course early. You can try to change a family history of fat. Adults, teens, and kids all have to eat right and stay active to be fit and healthy. You know the basics of getting and staying fit. They're the same for everyone, big and small. Kids are individuals, just like adults, and they have individual preferences for certain foods and certain types of activities. To get them to eat right and exercise more, you have to help them design their own individual plans for healthy eating and exercise. Here are some kid-size nutrition and fitness tips:

➤ Encourage kids to participate in active play and sports-like activities.

➤ Exercise with your children. Develop a routine you can all follow at least a few times a week.

➤ Teach children about good nutrition by setting a good example at family dinners.

➤ Introduce children to as many new foods as possible. You're bound to hit on at least a few healthy foods they'll like.

➤ Take the kids food shopping. Ask them to pick out fruits and vegetables they want to eat.

➤ Find creative ways to get your kids to eat vegetables. For example, add grated carrots to homemade muffins, ground meat mixtures, and peanut butter sandwiches. Combine chopped fresh tomatoes and sweet peppers with a jar of salsa to give the dip a nutrition boost.

➤ Kids like to eat foods they cook themselves. Teach them how to cook whole-grain muffins, simple vegetable dishes, and other healthful foods.

➤ Don't be afraid to make rules. No eating and TV watching at the same time!

> **Guru's Corner**
> "Kids respond best to fitness when it's pure fun. They're motivated by success so be sure to praise your kids for even the smallest physical accomplishment."
>
> —Roxie W. Greene, ACE Certified Group Fitness Instructor and owner of KIDZPLAY in Greer, South Carolina

The Least You Need to Know

➤ Everyone hits a weight plateau at some point and stops losing weight. You have to have patience and faith because no matter how long it lasts, the plateau will eventually break and you'll start losing again.

➤ To maintain a healthy weight, you pretty much have to do the same things you did to get to it.

➤ You might be able to help your kids avoid going through a lot of what you went through to lose weight by teaching them about good nutrition and fitness early.

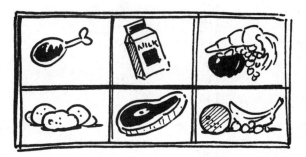

Calorie and Fat Chart for Selected Foods

Breads, Cereals, and Grain Foods

Food	Amount	Calories	Fat (in Grams)
Breads and Crackers			
Bagel	3-inch	163	1
Biscuit	1 small	105	5
Bread, Italian	1 slice	85	0
Bread, white	1 slice	75	1
Bread, whole wheat	1 slice	67	2
Bread, pumpernickel	1 slice	82	1
Cracker, saltine, multi-grain	5	60	2
Cracker, graham, low-fat	2 whole	110	2
Cracker, Ry-Krisp, plain	1 whole	84	0
Muffin, bran	1 small	112	5
Muffin, corn	1 small	125	4
Muffin, English	1 whole	133	1
Pancake	1 small	60	2
Roll, hard	1	155	2

Breads, Cereals, and Grain Foods   Continued

Food	Amount	Calories	Fat (in Grams)
Cereals			
Bran flakes	1 cup	135	1
Cheerios	1 cup	110	2
Corn Chex	1 cup	111	0
Crispy rice	1 cup	110	0
Farina, cooked	1 cup	117	0
Grape Nuts	⅓ cup	136	0
Granola, low-fat	⅓ cup	110	2
Oat Bran, cooked	1 cup	88	2
Oatmeal, cooked	1 cup	150	3
Puffed rice, plain	1 cup	50	0
Raisin Bran	1 cup	174	1
Shredded Wheat	1 biscuit	80	0
Total	1 cup	100	1
Wheatena, cooked	1 cup	150	1
Wheaties	1 cup	101	1
Grains			
Barley, cooked	1 cup	195	1
Bulgur, cooked	1 cup	150	0
Couscous, cooked	1 cup	200	0
Macaroni, cooked	1 cup	183	1
Noodles, cooked	1 cup	213	2
Popcorn, plain, air-popped	1 cup	25	0
Pretzel stick, small thin	1	1	0
Pretzel twist, thin	1	24	0
Rice cake, regular	1	35	0
Rice, brown, cooked	1 cup	216	2
Rice, white, cooked	1 cup	264	1
Wheat germ, toasted	2 Tbsp.	54	2
Wheat bran	2 Tbsp.	15	0

Fruit

Food	Amount	Calories	Fat (in Grams)
Apple, medium	1	81	1
Applesauce, unsweetened	½ cup	53	0
Apple juice	1 cup	116	0
Apricot	1	17	0
Apricot, dried	¼ cup	77	0
Banana, medium	1	105	1
Blueberries	1 cup	81	1
Cranberry juice cocktail	1 cup	144	0
Cranberry sauce, sweetened	¼ cup	105	0
Grapefruit	½	37	0
Kiwi	1	45	0
Melon, honeydew cubes	1 cup	60	0
Nectarine	1	67	1
Orange, medium	1	62	1
Orange juice, fresh	1 cup	112	1
Papaya, cut up	1 cup	55	0
Peach	1	37	0
Pear, Bartlett	1	98	1
Pineapple, cut up	1 cup	76	1
Plum	1	36	0
Prunes, stewed	½ cup	106	0
Raisins	¼ cup	109	1
Raspberries	1 cup	60	1
Rhubarb, cut up	1 cup	26	0
Strawberries	1 cup	45	1
Tangerine	1	37	0
Watermelon, cut up	1 cup	51	1

Vegetables

Food	Amount	Calories	Fat (in Grams)
Asparagus, cooked	½ cup	22	0
Beans, green, cooked	½ cup	22	0
Beets, cooked, sliced	½ cup	26	0

continues

Vegetables   Continued

Food	Amount	Calories	Fat (in Grams)
Broccoli, cooked	½ cup	23	0
Brussels sprouts, cooked	½ cup	30	0
Cabbage, raw, shredded	1 cup	16	0
Carrot, whole	1 medium	31	0
Cauliflower, cooked	½ cup	15	0
Celery, raw	1 stalk	6	0
Eggplant, cooked	½ cup	23	0
Kale, cooked	½ cup	21	0
Lettuce, raw, chopped	1 cup	10	0
Mushrooms, sliced, cooked	½ cup	21	0
Okra, cooked	½ cup	34	0
Onion, yellow, cooked	½ cup	30	0
Onion, green, raw	½ cup	13	0
Peas, green, cooked from frozen	½ cup	63	0
Pepper, green, chopped, cooked	½ cup	12	0
Potato, white, baked, with skin	1 medium	220	0
Potato, sweet, baked, peeled	1 medium	118	0
Radishes, raw	10	7	0
Spinach, raw	1 cup	12	0
Spinach, cooked	½ cup	20	0
Squash, zucchini, cooked	½ cup	15	0
Squash, acorn, cooked, mashed	½ cup	42	0
Tomato	1	24	0
Tomato, chopped	½ cup	18	0

Milk and Dairy Products

Food	Amount	Calories	Fat (in Grams)
Cheese			
American	1 oz.	106	9
Blue	1 oz.	100	8
Brie	1 oz.	95	8
Cheddar	1 oz.	114	9

Food	Amount	Calories	Fat (in Grams)
Cheese			
Cottage, 1 percent low-fat	1 cup	164	2
Cottage, regular	1 cup	234	10
Feta	1 oz.	75	6
Gouda	1 oz.	101	8
Monterey Jack	1 oz.	106	9
Muenster	1 oz.	104	9
Parmesan, grated	1 oz.	129	9
Provolone	1 oz.	100	8
Ricotta, part-skim	½ cup	170	10
Ricotta, whole milk	½ cup	214	16
Romano	1 oz.	110	8
Swiss	1 oz.	107	8
Milk			
Skim	1 cup	90	1
1 percent low-fat	1 cup	102	3
2 percent	1 cup	121	5
Whole	1 cup	150	8
Buttermilk	1 cup	99	2
Yogurt			
Plain, nonfat	1 cup	127	trace
Plain, low-fat	1 cup	144	4
Plain, whole	1 cup	139	7

Meat, Poultry, Seafood, and Meat Substitutes*

Food	Amount	Calories	Fat (in Grams)
Meat			
Bacon, cooked	1 slice	36	3
Beef, flank steak, cooked	3 oz.	176	9
Beef, ground, lean	3 oz.	230	15
Beef, bottom round, cooked	3 oz.	178	7
Beef, sirloin, cooked	3 oz.	165	6

continues

Meat, Poultry, Seafood, and Meat Substitutes*   Continued

Food	Amount	Calories	Fat (in Grams)
Meat			
Beef, top round, cooked	3 oz.	153	4
Ham, cured, cooked	3 oz.	140	6.5
Lamb, arm, cooked	3 oz.	173	9
Lamb, leg, cooked	3 oz.	162	7
Lamb, shank, cooked	3 oz.	153	6
Pork, center loin, cooked	3 oz.	204	11
Pork, tenderloin, roasted, lean	3 oz.	141	4
Veal, arm, cooked	3 oz.	139	5
Veal, rib, cooked	3 oz.	150	6
Veal, top round, cooked	3 oz.	128	3
Poultry			
Chicken, white meat, cooked	3 oz.	142	3
Chicken, drumstick, cooked	3 oz.	151	5
Chicken, thigh, cooked	3 oz.	163	7
Turkey, white meat, cooked	3 oz.	115	1
Turkey, dark meat, cooked	3 oz.	137	4
Egg, whole, large	1	75	5
Egg, white, large	1	16	0
Egg, yolk, large	1	59	5
Seafood			
Catfish, cooked	3 oz.	129	7
Cod, cooked	3 oz.	89	1
Flounder, cooked	3 oz.	99	1
Halibut, cooked	3 oz.	119	3
Mackerel, cooked	3 oz.	171	9
Monkfish, cooked	3 oz.	82	2
Orange roughy, cooked	3 oz.	75	1
Salmon			
Atlantic, cooked	3 oz.	175	11
Coho, cooked	3 oz.	151	7
Salmon, pink, canned	3 oz.	114	5
Snapper, cooked	3 oz.	109	2
Surimi (imitation seafood)	3 oz.	84	1

Food	Amount	Calories	Fat (in Grams)
Seafood			
Swordfish, cooked	3 oz.	132	4
Trout, rainbow, cooked	3 oz.	128	5
Tuna, fresh, cooked	3 oz.	156	5
Tuna, white, canned in water	3 oz.	90	1
Shellfish			
Clams, canned, drained	3 oz.	126	2
Crab, king, cooked	3 oz.	82	1
Lobster, cooked	3 oz.	84	1
Oysters, cooked	3 oz.	116	4
Scallops, cooked	3 oz.	75	1
Shrimp, cooked	3 oz.	84	1

Note: 4 ounces raw meat, poultry or seafood generally yields 3 ounces cooked. Meat values are for lean portion only.

Legumes

Food	Amount	Calories	Fat (in Grams)
Beans, lima, cooked	½ cup	94	0
Beans, black, cooked	½ cup	125	1
Beans, garbanzo, cooked	½ cup	143	1
Beans, navy, cooked	½ cup	129	1
Beans, pinto, cooked	½ cup	117	0
Lentils, cooked	½ cup	115	0
Split peas, cooked	½ cup	116	0
Tofu	3 oz.	88	6

Nuts and Seeds

Food	Amount	Calories	Fat (in Grams)
Brazil	¼ cup	230	29
Cashew, dry roasted	¼ cup	197	16
Macadamia, oil roasted	¼ cup	240	26
Peanuts, oil roasted	¼ cup	210	18

continues

Nuts and Seeds   Continued

Food	Amount	Calories	Fat (in Grams)
Peanut butter, smooth	1 Tbsp.	94	8
Pistachio, dry roasted	¼ cup	185	16
Pumpkin seeds, roasted	¼ cup	72	3
Sunflower seeds, oil roasted	¼ cup	208	20
Walnuts, chopped	¼ cup	190	18

Fats and Oils

Food	Amount	Calories	Fat (in Grams)
Butter	1 Tbsp.	102	12
Margarine	1 Tbsp.	102	11
Mayonnaise	1 Tbsp.	99	11
Mayonnaise, low calorie	1 Tbsp.	40	4
Oil, corn	1 Tbsp.	120	14
Oil, olive	1 Tbsp.	120	14
Salad dressing			
Blue cheese, regular	1 Tbsp.	77	8
Blue cheese, low calorie	1 Tbsp.	10	1
French, regular	1 Tbsp.	67	6
French, low calorie	1 Tbsp.	22	1
Italian, regular	1 Tbsp.	69	7
Italian, low calorie	1 Tbsp.	16	2
Thousand Island, regular	1 Tbsp.	59	6
Thousand Island, low calorie	1 Tbsp.	24	2
Vegetable oil cooking spray	1 spritz	1–7	0–1

The sources for all the nutrition information are the U.S. Department of Agriculture and individual food manufacturers.

Note: Grams of fat are rounded off to the nearest tenth. Calories and fat values for similar foods may vary widely, depending on the brand you use.

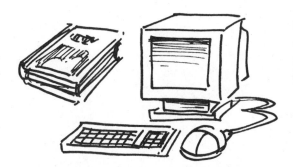

Your Best Resources

Organizations to Contact for Information and Support

American Anorexia/Bulimia Association
165 W. 46th St.
Suite 1108
New York, NY 10036
(212) 575-6200

American Council on Exercise
5820 Oberlin Drive, Suite 102
San Diego, CA 92121
(800) 529-8227
Web site: http://www.acefitness.org

American Dietetic Association
National Center for Nutrition and Dietetics
216 West Jackson Blvd.
Chicago, IL 60606-6995
(800) 366-1655 (automated information line)
(900) 225-5267 (to speak with a registered dietitian; $1.95 first minute; $0.95 each additional minute)
Web site: http://www.eatright.org

American Heart Association
National Center
7272 Greenville Ave.
Dallas, TX 75231-4596
(800) 242-8721 (for local chapters)
Web site: http://207.211.141.25

American Society for Bariatric Physicians
5600 S. Quebec St.
Suite 109-A
Englewood, CO 80111
(303) 779-4833

Food and Nutrition Information Center
U.S. Department of Agriculture
National Agricultural Library
10301 Baltimore Blvd.
Room 304
Beltsville, MD 20725-2351
(301) 504-5719

National Association to Advance Fat Acceptance
P.O. Box 188620
Sacramento, CA 95818
(916) 558-6880

Nutrition Information Service
University of Alabama at Birmingham
Webb Building, Room 447
UAB Station
Birmingham, AL 35294
(800) 231-DIET

Weight-Control Information Network (WIN)
National Institutes of Health
National Institute of Diabetes and Digestive and Kidney Diseases
1 Win Way
Bethesda, MD 20892-3665
(800) 946-8098
Web site: http://www.niddk.nih.gov/nutritiondocs.html

Internet Resources

Healthy Weight
http://healthyweight.com

CyberDiet
http://cyberdiet.com

Health Vision Diet & Weight Loss/Fitness Home Page
http://www1.mhv.net./~donn/diet.html

Reading List

Books

ACSM Fitness Book
American College of Sports Medicine (Leisure Press, 1992)

The American Dietetic Association's Complete Food & Nutrition Guide
by Roberta Larson Duyff, M.S., R.D., CFCS (Chronimed Publishing, 1996)

The Tufts University Guide to Total Nutrition
by Stanley Gershoff, Ph.D., and the editors of the Tufts University Diet & Nutrition
Letter, 2nd Ed. (Harper Collins, 1996)

If Your Child Is Overweight: A Guide for Parents
by Susan M. Kosharek (The American Dietetic Association, 1993)

A Substance Called Food
by Gloria Arenson (McGraw-Hill, 1989)

Full Lives: Women Who Have Freed Themselves from Food & Weight Obsession
by Lindsey Hall (Gürze Books, 1993)

Hugs from the Refrigerator
by James McClernan, Ed.D. (Westport Publishers, 1994)

Just the Weigh You Are: How to Be Fit and Healthy, Whatever Your Size
by Steven Jonas, M.D., and Linda Konner (Houghton Mifflin/Chapters 1997)

Like Mother, Like Daughter
by Debra Waterhouse, M.P.H., R.D. (Hyperion, 1997)

Outsmarting the Female Fat Cell
by Debra Waterhouse, M.P.H., R.D. (Warner Books, 1993)

Smart Exercise
by Covert Bailey (Houghton Mifflin, 1994)

The Supermarket Nutrition Counter
by Annette B. Natow, Ph.D., R.D., and Jo-Ann Heslin, M.A., R.D. (Pocket Books, 1997)

The Thin Books
by Jeane Eddy Westin (Hazelden, 1996)

Thin for Life
by Anne Fletcher, M.S., R.D. (Houghton Mifflin/Chapters)

Eating Thin for Life
by Anne Fletcher, M.S., R.D. (Houghton Mifflin/Chapters)

Cookbooks

Lighter, Quicker, Better
by Richard Sax and Marie Simmons (William Morrow, 1995)

Healthy Homestyle Cooking
by Evelyn Tribole, M.S., R.D. (Rodale Press, 1994)

Moosewood Restaurant's Low-Fat Favorites
(Clarkson Potter, 1996)

Sweetie Pie: The Richard Simmons Private Collection of Dazzling Desserts
(GT Publishing, 1997)

Weight Watchers Versatile Vegetarian
(Macmillan, 1997)

Prevention's The Healthy Cook
(Rodale Press, 1997)

Healthy Cooking for Two (or Just You)
by Frances Price, R.D. (Rodale Press, 1995)

Note: To order Rodale Press books, call (800) 848-4735.

Newsletters

Consumer Reports on Health
Box 56356
Boulder, CO 80322-6356
(800) 234-5384

Environmental Nutrition
P.O. Box 420235
Palm Coast, FL 32142-0451
(800) 829-5384

Mayo Clinic Health Letter
Subscription Services
P.O. Box 53889
Boulder, CO 80322-3889
(800) 333-9037

Tufts University Diet & Nutrition Letter
P.O. Box 57857
Boulder, CO 80322-7857
(800) 274-7581

Nutrition Action Health Letter
Center for Science in the Public Interest
Suite 300
Washington, DC 20009
(800) 237-4874

University of California at Berkeley Wellness Letter
Health Letter Associates
P.O. Box 420235
Palm Coast, FL 32142
(800) 829-9080

Magazines

Cooking Light
(800) 336-0125

Going Bonkers? The Magazine for Overcoming Stress
(800) 777-1999

Eating Well
(800) 678-0541

Shape, Living Fit, and *Men's Fitness*
(800) 998-0731

Index

Symbols

1,600 Calorie Open Exchange Checklist, 246

A

abs classes, 185
acesulfame potassium (artificial sweetener), 122
activities
    Alternate Activities Record, 211
    selecting for exercise, 174-176
addiction to food, 65
adult-onset diabetes, 9
advice, locating 53
aerobic exercise, 177-178, 195-197
    cool-downs, 197
    training heart rate, 196-197
    warm-ups, 196
Aerobics and Fitness Association of America, 198
aerobics classes, types of, 185
affirmations, 232-233
    writing, 234
alcoholic drinks, 168-169
Alternate Activities Record, 211
alternative weight loss methods
    fasting, 56-57
    meditation, 56
alternatives
    for desserts, 271-272
        baking substitutions, 272
        fruit, 272
    to eating habits, 113
American Anorexia/Bulimia Association, 291
American Council on Exercise, 198, 291
American Dietetic Association, 291
American Heart Association, 292
American Society for Bariatric Physicians, 292
amino acids, 122
    for vegetarians, 123-124
    sources, 123
anaerobic exercise, 177-178
anorexia nervosa, 42
appetite suppressants, see diet pills
appetites, 209
    compared to hunger, 209
    emotional, 209-211
apples, Quickie "Baked" Apple recipe, 267
artificial sweeteners, 121-122
aspartame (artificial sweetener), 121
assessment, personal questions, 71-72
    eating habits, 72-73
    lifestyle changes, 72
attitudes
    food avoidance, 214-215
    patience, 215
    toward losing weight, 68-71, 82
    visualization techniques, 214
avoiding
    certain foods, 214-215
    trigger situations, 82

B

baking, food substitutions in desserts, 272
balanced meals, planning, 154
balancing calories with exercise, 162-163
ballroom dancing (U.S. Amateur Ballroom Dancers Association), 191
bamboo steamers, 258
basal metabolism, 118
    rate, 105
basic kitchen equipment, 259
BBQ (barbeque), Janine D'Amato's Vegetarian BBQ-on-a-Bun recipe, 265
beans, calorie/fat grams chart, 289
behavior, see habits
behavior modification, 212-214
behavioral goals, 85
Beverly Hills Diet, 49
binge eating disorder, 43
blaming yourself for weight gain, 21, 221-222
BMI (body mass index) chart, 16-17
body
    apple-shaped, 17
    lean body mass, 179
    metabolism, 118-119
    minimum calories needed, 104
    pear-shaped, 17
    starvation mode, 20, 64
body fat, measuring percentage, 4

body mass index (BMI) chart, 16-17
body sculpting classes, 185
books, bibliographic information, 293-294
box aerobics classes, 185
brain chemicals, effect on eating habits, 29
breads, calorie/fat grams chart, 283
breads, cereals, rice, and pasta food group, 141-142
breaking eating habits, 99-101
bulimia, 42-43
burning calories
    body metabolism, 118-119
    during exercise, 189
    during walking, 202
    sex, 90
    to lose one pound, 21
buying
    exercise equipment, 192
    exercise videos, 193

C

Cabbage Soup diet, 50
caffeine, effect on exercise, 191
calculating fat intake, 119, 126-127
calorie chart
    breads, 283
    cereals, 284
    cheese, 286-287
    fats and oils, 290
    fruit, 285
    grains, 284
    legumes, 289
    meat, 287-288
    milk, 287
    nuts and seeds, 289-290
    poultry, 288
    seafood, 288-289
    vegetables, 285-286
    yogurt, 287
calorie free, defined, 252
calories, 119-120
    alcoholic drinks, 168-169
    balanced meals, 154
    balancing with exercise, 162-163
    body metabolism, 118-119

burning
    during exercise, 189
    during walking, 202
    sex, 90
    to lose one pound, 21
counting, 104
    formulas for, 104-106
    menu plans, 106-111
    mixed messages about, 51-52
    setting ranges, 106
fat intake, calculating, 126-127
Cambridge diet, 49
cancer, 9
canned food, shopping for, 255-256
carbohydrate-based fat substitutes, 127
carbohydrates, 120
    artificial sweeteners, 121-122
    complex, 121
    mixed messages about, 52-53
    simple, 120-121
cardio-step aerobics classes, 185
cereals, calorie/fat grams chart, 284
Champagne diet, 49
changing habits, 212, 231
    affirmations, 232-234
    behavior modification, 212-214
    positive thoughts, 231-232
cheese, calorie/fat grams chart, 286-287
chicken
    Chicken Cutlets with Lemon and Basil recipe, 263-264
    shopping for, 254
Chicken Cutlets with Lemon and Basil recipe, 263-264
children
    calorie-restricted diets, 50
    childhood habits, effect on losing weight, 18-19
    healthy eating habits, encouraging, 281
    teaching healthy eating habits, 27
Chocolate Lover's Diet, 48
cholesterol, reducing, 165

classes (health clubs), selecting, 185
cod, Orange-Soy Glazed Cod Steaks recipe, 264-265
Collage Video, exercise videos, 193
commercial weight-loss programs, 59-61
    Diet Center, 63
    evaluating, 66
    Jenny Craig, 62
    joining multiple times, 63
    Nutri-System, 62
    Weight Watchers, 61-62
commitment to weight loss, 207-208
complex carbohydrates, 121
compulsive overeating, 217
    questionnaire, 218
    solutions for, 218-219
constructive procrastination, 221
Consumer Reports on Health Newsletter, 294
contemplation stage, 83
convenience food, 274-275
cookbooks, 294
cooking
    with basic kitchen equipment, 259
    with microwave ovens, 257-258
    with steamers, 258
    see also food; nutrition
cool-down exercises, 197
coping with stress, 224-225
counselors, personal assessment questions, 71-72
    eating habits, 72-73
    lifestyle changes, 72
counting calories, 104
    formulas for, 104-106
    menu plans, 106-111
    mixed messages about, 51-52
    setting ranges, 106
CPE gene, 28
Craig, Jenny, 62
cravings, solutions for, 270
Creamy Vegetable Soup recipe, 262
cross-training, 200
cutlery, 258-259
CyberDiet Web site, 293

D

Daily Value information on Nutrition Facts labels, 250
dairy products
    calorie/fat grams chart, 286-287
    shopping for, 253
dancing, 190-191
depression and binge eating disorder, 43
desserts
    healthy alternatives for, 271-272
        baking substitutions, 272
        fruit, 272
    recipes for, 267
diabetes, 9
diary, *see* food diary
Diet Center, commercial weight-loss program, 63
diet pills
    health hazards, 55
    over-the-counter, 55
    prescription, 56
Diet Revolution, 48
Dietary Guidelines for Americans, 159-160
    alcoholic drinks, 168-169
    balancing calories and exercise, 162-163
    fat intake, reducing, 164-165
    grains, fruits, and vegetables, 163-164
    salt, reducing, 166-167
    sugar, reducing, 165-166
    variety of food, 160-162
dietary supplements, *see* supplements
diets, *see also* food; nutrition
    and children, 50
    commercial weight-loss programs, 59-61
        Diet Center, 63
        evaluating, 66
        Jenny Craig, 62
        joining multiple times, 63
        Nutri-System, 62
        Weight Watchers, 61-62
    counting calories, mixed messages, 51-52

eating plans
    open exchange plan, 238, 245-247
    pick-a-meal plan, 238, 243-245
    selecting, 238-239
    straight menu plan, 238-242
evaluating, 54-55
expert advice, where to get, 53
fad diets, 20
    and starvation mode, 20
    dangers of, 49
high protein, 52
losing weight with, 8
low-fat, 51
mixed messages about, 50-51
    carbohydrates, 52-53
    counting calories, 51-52
    high protein diets, 52
    low-fat diets, 51
modified fasts, 63-64
reasons for failure, 22-23
types of, 48-50
yo-yo dieting, 10-11
diuretics, 55
DNA (deoxyribonucleic acid), 28
do-it-yourself plans, 75
    evaluation questions, 77
    support for, 76-77
dopamine, 29
drinks
    alcoholic, 168-169
    water, 132
        alternatives, 132-133
        during exercise, 176-177
        when to drink, 133

E

Eat More, Weigh Less, 50
eating, *see* food; nutrition
eating disorders
    anorexia nervosa, 42
    binge eating disorder, 43
    bulimia, 42-43
    medical consequences of, 43
    treatment for, 43-44
eating habits, 23
    alternatives to, 113
    and hunger, 208-209

appetites, 209
at parties, 275
at restaurants, 274
avoiding trigger situations, 82
brain chemicals' effect, 29
breaking, 99-101
changing, behavior modification, 212-214
compulsive overeating, 217
    questionnaire, 218
    solutions for, 218-219
emotional appetites, 209-211
encouraging children in, 281
family influences on, 25-27
fast food, 274-275
food diary, 94
    categories in, 94-96
    how to use, 98-99
improving, 89-90
questions, 72-73
teaching children, 27
when traveling, 273
when to stop eating, 212
eating plans
    open exchange plan, 238, 245-247
    pick-a-meal plan, 238, 243-245
    selecting, 238-239
    straight menu plan, 238-242
emotional appetites, 209-211
emotional reactions
    compulsive overeating, 217
        questionnaire, 218
        solutions for, 218-219
    excuses, 220-222
        blaming yourself and others, 221-222
        procrastination, 220-221
    fear, 229
        of failure, 230
        of fat, 229
        of success, 229-230
        worksheet, 230
    perfectionism, 219-220
    self-esteem, 222-223
    stress, 223
        internal/external stressors, 223-224
        managing, 224-225
emotional responses
    expectations, 40-41
    guilt, 38-39
        reasons for, 39
        solutions for, 40

negative thoughts
 effect of, 36-37
  expecting perfection, 38
  solutions for, 37-38
 to weight gain, 21-22
emotions and brain chemicals'
 effect, 29
empty calorie food, 73
endorphins, 29
endurance, effect of exercise, 179
energy metabolism, 118-119
Environmental Nutrition
 Newsletter, 294
equipment (exercise), selecting,
 192
equipment for kitchen, 257
 basics, 259
 knives, 258-259
 microwave ovens, 257-258
 steamers, 258
essential amino acids, 123
etiquette at health clubs, 186
evaluating
 commercial weight-loss
  programs, 66
 diets, 54-55
 do-it-yourself weight loss, 77
excess weight, *see* overweight
 people
exchanges, *see* open exchange
 plan
excuses for not losing weight,
 21, 220-222
 blaming yourself and others,
  221-222
 procrastination, 220-221
exercise
 advantages of, 174
 aerobic, 195-197
  cool-downs, 197
  training heart rate,
   196-197
  warm-ups, 196
 balancing calories with,
  162-163
 burning calories, 189
 cross-training, 200
 dancing, 190-191
 equipment, selecting, 192
 Exercise Log, 202
 goals, 85
 health benefits, 177-179
 health clubs
  classes, selecting, 185
  etiquette, 186

  instructors, 185-186
  selecting, 183-184
 at home, 191-193
 increasing, 90
 lean body mass, 179
 motivation for, 176
 psychological benefits,
  178-179
 selecting activities, 174-176
 sports, 186
  golf, 187
  in-line skating, 188
  skiing, 188-189
  swimming, 187-188
  tennis, 187
 strength training,
  178-179, 197-199
 t'ai chi, 178
 types of, 177-178
 videos, selecting, 193
 walking
  burning calories, 202
  style of, 201-202
 warm-up, 181
 weather conditions, 176-177
 workout schedule, 180-181
 yoga, 178
Exercise Log, 202
expectations, 40-41
expert advice, 53
external stressors, 223-224

F

Facing Your Fears Worksheet,
 230
fad diets, 20
 and starvation mode, 20
 dangers of, 49
 examples of, 48-50
 high protein diets, 52
failure, fear of, 230
failure of diets, reasons for, 22-23
fair exchanges, open exchange
 meal plan, 247
fake fat, 127-128
family
 encouraging healthy eating
  habits, 281
 influences on weight gain,
  25-27
 support from, 30-31
fast food, 274-275

fasting, 56-57
 modified fasts, 63-64
fat, 125
 calorie/fat grams chart, 290
 fear of, 229
 gaining weight from, 127
 in meat, 253-254
 in poultry, 254
 saturated, reducing, 165
 substitutes, 127-128
 types of, 126
 see also body fat
fat cells, effect on losing
 weight, 19
fat free, defined, 252
fat grams chart
 breads, 283
 cereals, 284
 cheese, 286-287
 fats and oils, 290
 fruit, 285
 grains, 284
 legumes, 289
 meat, 287-288
 milk, 287
 nuts and seeds, 289-290
 poultry, 288
 seafood, 288-289
 vegetables, 285-286
 yogurt, 287
fat intake
 calculating, 119, 126-127
 low-fat diets, 51
 reducing, 164-165
fat soluble vitamins, 134
fat-based fat substitutes, 128
fat-free desserts, dangers of, 271
fats, oils, and sweets food group,
 141
fear
 of failure, 230
 of fat, 229
 of success, 229-230
 worksheet, 230
Ferguson, Sybil, Diet Center
 program, 63
fiber
 amount of, 131-132
 insoluble, 130
 soluble, 130-131
fish
 calorie/fat grams chart,
  288-289
 Orange-Soy Glazed Cod Steaks
  recipe, 264-265
 shopping for, 254-255

Fit for Life diet, 50
fitness
    children, encouraging, 281
    exercise
        advantages of, 174
        aerobic, 195-197
        burning calories, 189
        cool-downs, 197
        cross-training, 200
        dancing, 190-191
        equipment, selecting, 192
        Exercise Log, 202
        health benefits of, 177-179
        at home, 191-193
        lean body mass, 179
        motivation for, 176
        psychological benefits,
            178-179
        selecting activities, 174-176
        strength training,
            178-179, 197-199
        training heart rate,
            196-197
        types of, 177-178
        videos, selecting, 193
        walking, 201-202
        warm-ups, 196
        weather conditions,
            176-177
        workout schedule, 180-181
    health clubs
        classes, selecting, 185
        etiquette, 186
        instructors, 185-186
        selecting, 183-184
    healthy weight, 11
    sports, 186
        golf, 187
        in-line skating, 188
        skiing, 188-189
        swimming, 187-188
        tennis, 187
flexibility
    effect of exercise on, 179
    of open exchange meal plan,
        247
fluctuation in weight, 111
fluids, *see* drinks
FNIC (Food and Nutrition
    Information Center), 54
food
    appetites, 209
    avoiding certain foods,
        214-215
    calories, 119-120

carbohydrates, 120
    artificial sweeteners,
        121-122
    complex, 121
    mixed messages about,
        52-53
    simple, 120-121
    in commercial weight-loss
        programs, 60
cooking
    basic kitchen equipment,
        259
    with microwave ovens,
        257-258
    with steamers, 258
counting calories
    formulas for, 104-106
    menu plans, 106-111
    mixed messages about,
        51-52
    setting ranges, 106
cravings, solutions for, 270
desserts, healthy alternatives,
    271-272
Dietary Guidelines for
    Americans, 159-160
    alcoholic drinks, 168-169
    balancing calories and
        exercise, 162-163
    fat intake, reducing,
        164-165
    grains, fruits, and veg-
        etables, 163-164
    salt, reducing, 166-167
    sugar, reducing, 165-166
    variety of food, 160-162
diets
    evaluating, 54-55
    reasons for failure, 22-23
eating habits questions, 72-73
eating plans
    open exchange plan, 238,
        245-247
    pick-a-meal plan, 238,
        243-245
    selecting, 238-239
    straight menu plan,
        238-242
emotional appetites, 209-211
empty calorie food, 73
fad diets, 20
fat, 125
    calculating intake, 126-127
    fear of, 229
    gaining weight from, 127

substitutes, 127-128
    types of, 126
fiber
    amount of, 131-132
    insoluble, 130
    soluble, 130-131
goals, 85
high protein diets, 52
labels, meanings of terms, 252
low-fat diets, 51
low-fat substitutes, 268
mineral sources, 135, 160-162
Nutrition Facts labels, Daily
    Value information, 250
phytochemicals, 137
protein, 122
    for vegetarians, 123-124
    RDA (Recommended Daily
        Allowance), 124-125
    sources, 123
recipes
    desserts, 267
    main dishes, 263-265
    side dishes, 265-266
    soup, 262
    vinaigrette, 262-263
shopping for, 252
    canned food, 255-256
    cupboard stocking, 257
    dairy products, 253
    frozen foods, 255
    grains, 256
    meat, 253-254
    poultry, 254
    produce department, 253
    seafood, 254-255
skipping meals, 104
snacking, solutions for,
    270-271
substitutions in desserts, 272
sugar
    effect on teeth, 166
    sources of, 166
vitamin sources,
    134-135, 160-162
when to stop eating, 212
see also eating habits;
    nutrition
food addiction, 65
Food and Nutrition Information
    Center (FNIC), 54, 292
food diary, 94
    breaking bad eating habits,
        99-101

categories in, 94-96
how to use, 98-99
Food Frequency Question-
naire, 73
food pyramid, 140-141
balanced meals, 154
breads, cereals, rice, and pasta
food group, 141-142
fats, oils, and sweets food
group, 141
fruit food group, 141-142
meat, poultry, fish, dry beans,
eggs, and nuts food group,
141-143
milk, yogurt, and cheese food
group, 141-143
open exchange meal plan,
245-247
Pyramid Menu Plan, 157
serving sizes, 141-144
vegetable food group, 141-142
formulas
counting calories, 104-106
for healthy weight range, 14
fresh foods, 163-164
frozen foods, shopping for, 255
fruits
as dessert, 272
calorie/fat grams chart, 285
fresh, 163-164
Quickie "Baked" Apple recipe,
267
shopping for, 253
when to eat, 164
fruit food group, 141-142
funk aerobics classes, 185

G

gaining weight
compulsive overeating, 217
questionnaire, 218
solutions for, 218-219
differences among people, 21
emotional responses to, 21-22
family influences on, 25-27
from fat, 127
reasons for, 20
when extra pounds are okay,
17-18
yo-yo dieting, 10-11
Garlic and Herb Meat Rub recipe,
264

genetic studies, 28
glucose, 120
dangers of high protein
diets, 52
goals, 84
behavioral, 85
exercise, 85
food, 85
intermediate, 84
long-term, 84
patience, 215
psychological, 85
setting, 31-32
short-term, 84
types of, 85
very-short-term, 84
golf, 187
grains
calorie/fat grams chart, 284
fresh, 163-164
shopping for, 256
grams, 119
fat intake, calculating,
126-127
Grapefruit diet, 48
grocery shopping, 252
canned food, 255-256
dairy products, 253
food labels, meanings of
terms, 252
for cupboard stocking, 257
frozen foods, 255
grains, 256
meat department, 253-254
Nutrition Facts labels, Daily
Value information, 250
poultry, 254
produce department, 253
seafood, 254-255
group programs, *see* commercial
weight-loss programs
groups, *see* support groups
guilt, 38-39
reasons for, 39
solutions for, 40
gyms
classes, selecting, 185
etiquette, 186
instructors, 185-186
selecting, 183-184

H

habits, 207
changing, 212, 231
affirmations, 232-234
behavior modification,
212-214
positive thoughts, 231-232
commitment to weight loss,
207-208
eating habits, 23
and hunger, 208-209
appetites, 209
at parties, 275
at restaurants, 274
avoiding trigger situations,
82
brain chemicals' effect on,
29
breaking, 99-101
emotional appetites,
209-211
encouraging children, 281
family influences on, 25-27
fast food, 274-275
improving, 89-90
teaching children, 27
when traveling, 273
when to stop eating, 212
effect on losing weight, 18-19
lifestyle changes, 112-113
alternatives to eating, 113
rewards for losing weight,
114
Hacker's diet, 50
health clubs
classes, selecting, 185
etiquette, 186
instructors, 185-186
selecting, 183-184
health hazards
diet pills, 55
over-the-counter, 55
prescription, 56
fad diets, 49
fasting, 56-57
high protein diets, 52
laxatives, 55
modified fasts, 64
of obesity, 9-10
Health Management Resources,
64
Health Vision Diet & Weight
Loss/Fitness Home Page, 293

Healthtouch Online Web site, 44
healthy eating habits, *see* eating habits
healthy weight
  apple-shaped body compared to pear-shaped, 17
  counting calories
    formulas, 104-106
    menu plans, 106-111
    setting ranges, 106
  definition of, 4-6
  fitness level, 11
  maintenance, 279-280
  ranges for, 14-15, 86-87
    body mass index chart, 16-17
  role models for, 227-229
  when extra pounds are okay, 17-18
Healthy Weight Web site, 293
heart disease, 9
heart rate during aerobic exercise, 196-197
help, *see* resources
heredity, effect on losing weight, 18-19
high blood pressure, 9
high-protein diets, 52
high-low impact aerobics classes, 185
holidays, 275
hunger
  compared to appetites, 209
  and eating habits, 208-209
hypertension, 9

I

ideal weight, *see* healthy weight
improving
  eating habits, 89-90
  motivation for losing weight, 90-91
incentives, *see* motivation for losing weight
increasing exercise, 90
in-line skating, 188
insoluble fiber, 130
instructors at health clubs, 185-186
intermediate goals, 84
internal stressors, 223-224
iron sources, 135

J - K

Janine D'Amato's Vegetarian BBQ-on-a-Bun recipe, 265
Jenny Craig weight-management program, 62
Joseph, Dr. Robert, Chocolate Lover's Diet, 48
Katz, Harold, Nutri-System, 62
ketone bodies, 57
ketosis, 52
kids, *see* children
kitchen equipment, 257
  basics, 259
  knives, 258-259
  microwave ovens, 257-258
  steamers, 258

L

labels
  meanings of terms, 252
  Nutrition Facts labels, Daily Value information, 250
laxatives, dangers of, 55
lean body mass, 179
legumes, calorie/fat grams chart, 289
leptin, 28
lifestyle changes, 72, 112-113
  alternatives to eating, 113
  rewards for losing weight, 114
  weight maintenance, 280
liquids, *see* drinks
long-term goals, 84
losing weight
  alternative methods, 56
    fasting, 56-57
    meditation, 56
  attitude toward, 82
    food avoidance, 214-215
    patience, 215
    visualization techniques, 214
  commitment to, 207-208
  diet types, 48-50
  differences among people, 21
  difficulty of, 7-9
  do-it-yourself plans, 75
    evaluation questions, 77
    support for, 76-77
  effect of habits on, 18-19
  expectations, 40-41

expert advice, where to get, 53
fad diets, 20
finding information about, 23
goals, 31-32, 84-85
mixed messages about,
  carbohydrates, 52-53
  counting calories, 51-52
  high protein diets, 52
  low fat diets, 51
motivation for, 68, 112-113
  alternative activities to eating, 113
  rewards, 114
number/size of fat cells, 19
personal assessment questions, 71-72
  eating habits, 72-73
  lifestyle changes, 72
personal attitude toward, 68-72
preparation for, 81-82
  eating habits, tips for improving, 89-90
  exercise tips, 90
  motivation, 90-91
  stages of change, 82-84
resources
  books, 293-294
  magazines, 295
  newsletters, 294-295
  organizations, 291-292
successful strategies for, 12
support for, 230-231
support from family and friends, 30-31
to-do list, 33
yo-yo dieting, 10-11
low calorie, defined, 252
low-fat diets, 51
low saturated fat, defined, 252
low-fat food substitutes, 268
lowering fat intake, 164-165

M

magazines, reference resources, 295
main dish recipes, 263-265
maintaining healthy weight, 279-280
maintenance stage, 83
managing stress, 224-225
Mayo Clinic Health Letter, 295
Mayo diet, 48

meals
  balanced, planning, 154
  planning (Pyramid Menu
    Plan), 157
  skipping, 104
measuring
  percentage of body fat, 4
  waist-to-hip ratio, 17
meat
  calorie/fat grams chart,
    287-288
  Garlic and Herb Meat Rub
    recipe, 264
  shopping for, 253-254
meat, poultry, fish, dry beans,
  eggs, and nuts food group,
  141-143
medical consequences of eating
  disorders, 43
medications, *see* pills
Medifast, 64
meditation, 56
  t'ai chi, 178
  yoga, 178
men compared to women in
  weight loss, 19
menus
  balanced meals, 154
  counting calories, 106-111
  open exchange plan, 238,
    245-247
  pick-a-meal plan, 238,
    243-245
  straight menu plan, 238-242
metabolism, 118-119
  minimum calories needed,
    104
Metrical, 48
microwave ovens, 257-258
milk, calorie/fat grams chart,
  253, 287
milk, yogurt, and cheese food
  group, 141-143
minerals, 133-135
  sources of, 135, 160-162
  supplements, 136-137
minimum calories needed, 104
modified fasts, 63-64
monounsaturated fat, 126
moods and brain chemicals, 29
motivation
  for exercise, 176
  for losing weight, 68, 112-113
    alternatives to eating, 113
    improving, 90-91

rewards, 114
for weight maintenance, 280
muscles
  lean body mass, 179
  strength training, 197-199
  testing strength, 198-199

N

National Association to Advance
  Fat Acceptance, 292
National Eating Disorders
  Organization (NEDO), 44
National Institute of Mental
  Health, 44
negative stress, 223
negative thoughts
  effect of, 36-37
  expecting perfection, 38
  solutions for, 37-38
neurons, 29
neurotransmitters, 29
newsletter resources, 294-295
NIDDM (non-insulin dependent
  diabetes mellitus), 9
Nidetch, Jean, Weight
  Watchers, 61
no added sugars, defined, 252
non-insulin dependent diabetes
  mellitus (NIDDM), 9
nonaerobic exercise, 177-178
NutraSweet, 121
Nutri-System, 62
nutrition
  calorie/fat grams chart
    breads, 283
    cereals, 284
    cheese, 286-287
    fats and oils, 290
    fruit, 285
    grains, 284
    legumes, 289
    meat, 287-288
    milk, 287
    nuts and seeds, 289-290
    poultry, 288
    seafood, 288-289
    vegetables, 285-286
    yogurt, 287
  calories, 119-120
  carbohydrates, 120
    artificial sweeteners,
      121-122
    complex, 121

mixed messages about,
  52-53
simple, 120-121
cholesterol, reducing, 165
counting calories, 104
  formulas for, 104-106
  menu plans, 106-111
  mixed messages about,
    51-52
  setting ranges, 106
Dietary Guidelines for
  Americans, 159-160
  alcoholic drinks, 168-169
  balancing calories and
    exercise, 162-163
  fat intake, reducing,
    164-165
  grains, fruits, and veg-
    etables, 163-164
  salt, reducing, 166-167
  sugar, reducing, 165-166
  variety of food, 160-162
diets
  evaluating, 54-55
  reasons for failure, 22-23
eating habits questions, 72-73
eating plans
  open exchange plan, 238,
    245-247
  pick-a-meal plan, 238,
    243-245
  selecting, 238-239
  straight menu plan,
    238-242
empty-calorie food, 73
for exercise, 200
fad diets, 20
fat, 125
  calculating intake, 126-127
  fear of, 229
  gaining weight from, 127
  substitutes, 127-128
  types of, 126
fiber
  amount of, 131-132
  insoluble, 130
  soluble, 130-131
food pyramid, 140-141
  balanced meals, 154
  breads, cereals, rice, and
    pasta food group,
    141-142
  fats, oils, and sweets food
    group, 141
  fruit food group, 141-142

meat, poultry, fish, dry beans, eggs, and nuts food group, 141-143
milk, yogurt, and cheese food group, 141-143
Pyramid Menu Plan, 157
serving sizes, 141-144
vegetable food group, 141-142
goals, 85
high protein diets, 52
low-fat diets, 51
low-fat food substitutes, 268
metabolism, 118-119
minerals, 133-135
phytochemicals, 137
protein, 122
RDA (Recommended Daily Allowance), 124-125
sources, 123
for vegetarians, 123-124
RDAs (Recommended Dietary Allowances), 54
skipping meals, 104
sugar
effect on teeth, 166
sources, 166
supplements, 136-137
vitamins, 133-135
water
alternatives to, 132-133
when to drink, 133
see also food
Nutrition Action Health Letter newsletter, 295
Nutrition Facts labels, Daily Value information, 250
Nutrition Information Service, 292
nuts, calorie/fat grams chart, 289-290

O

OA (Overeaters Anonymous), 65
OB gene, 28
obesity
definition, 4-6
genetic studies, 28
health hazards, 9-10
prescription diet pills, 56
oils, calorie/fat grams chart, 290
Olean, 128
Olestra, 128

open exchange plan, 238, 245-247
Optifast, 64
Orange-Soy Glazed Cod Steaks recipe, 264-265
Ornish, Dr. Dean, *Eat More, Weigh Less*, 50
over-the-counter diet pills, 55
Overeaters Anonymous (OA), 65
overweight people
definition of, 4-6
differences among, 21
family influences on, 25-27
fitness level, 11
health hazards, 9-10
healthy weight
body mass index chart, 16-17
ranges for, 14-15
percentages by state, 5-6
reasons for, 7, 20
habits learned in childhood, 18-19
number/size of fat cells, 19
support from family and friends, 30-31
when extra pounds are okay, 17-18

P

pasta, 256
percentage of body fat, measuring, 4
percentage of overweight people, state-by-state chart, 5-6
perfection, expecting, 38
perfectionism, 219-220
personal assessment questions, 71-72
eating habits, 72-73
lifestyle changes, 72
personal attitude toward losing weight, 68-71
personal trainers, 198
phenylpropanolamine (PPA), 55
phytochemicals, 137
pick-a-meal plan, 238, 243-245
pills
diet pills
health hazards, 55
over-the-counter, 55
prescription, 56
vitamin and mineral supplements, 136-137

planning
balanced meals, 154
meals (Pyramid Menu Plan), 157
plans
do-it-yourself, 75
evaluation questions, 77
support for, 76-77
eating plans
open exchange plan, 238, 245-247
pick-a-meal plan, 238, 243-245
selecting, 238-239
straight menu plan, 238-242
plateaus (weight), solutions, 277-279
polyunsaturated fat, 126
positive stress, 223
positive thoughts, 37-38, 231-232
Positive Thoughts Worksheet, 232
poultry
calorie/fat grams chart, 288
Chicken Cutlets with Lemon and Basil recipe, 263-264
shopping for, 254
PPA (phenylpropanolamine), 55
precontemplation stage, 83
preparation stage, 83
preparation for losing weight, 81-82
eating habits, tips for improving, 89-90
exercise tips, 90
motivation, 90-91
stages of change, 82-84
prescription diet pills, 56
Pritikin Plan, 49
procrastination, 220-221
produce department, 253
programs, *see* commercial weight-loss programs
protein, 122
high-protein diets, 52
RDA (Recommended Daily Allowance), 124-125
sources, 123
for vegetarians, 123-124
protein-based fat substitutes, 127
psychological benefits of exercise, 178-179
psychological goals, 85
pyramid, *see* food pyramid
Pyramid Menu Plan, 157

Q - R

Quickie "Baked" Apple recipe, 267

Rails-to-Trails Conservancy, 201
ranges for healthy weight, 14-15, 86-87
   body mass index chart, 16-17
RDA (Recommended Daily Allowance) of protein, 124-125
RDAs (Recommended Dietary Allowances), 54
reasons for being overweight, 7
recipes
   desserts, 267
   main dishes, 263-265
   side dishes, 265-266
   soup, 262
   vinaigrette, 262-263
recording
   eating habits in food diary, 94-99
   weight loss, 111-112
reduced calorie, defined, 252
reduced fat, defined 252
reduced saturated fat, defined, 252
reduced sugar, defined, 252
reducing
   cholesterol, 165
   fat intake, 164-165
   salt intake, 166-167
   stress, 224-225
   sugar intake, 165-166
removing skin from poultry, 254
resources for information
   books, 293-294
   magazines, 295
   newsletters, 294-295
   organizations, 291-292
   weight loss support, 230-231
restaurants, eating at, 274
resting metabolic rate, 105
rewards for losing weight, 114
rice, 256
role models, 227-229
Rotation Diet, 49
roughage, 130

S

saccharin (artificial sweetener), 122

salad
   bars, 253
   dressing, calorie/fat grams chart, 290
   vinaigrette recipe, 262-263
salad bars, 253
salad dressing, calorie/fat grams chart, 290
Salatrim, 128
salt, reducing intake, 166-167
saturated fat, 126
   reducing, 165
saturated fat free, defined, 252
scales, 111-112
Scarsdale Medical Diet, 49
scientific studies of obesity, 28
seafood
   calorie/fat grams chart, 288-289
   Orange-Soy Glazed Cod Steaks recipe, 264-265
   shopping for, 254-255
seeds, calorie/fat grams chart, 289-290
self-esteem, 222-223
self-love, 220
serotonin, 29
serving sizes for food, 141-144
   balanced meals, 154
   visualizing, 143-144
sex and burning calories, 90
shellfish
   calorie/fat grams chart, 289
   shopping, 254-255
shoes for walking, 201
shopping, *see* grocery shopping
Short Term Goal Organizer, 86
short-term goals, 84
side dishes, recipes, 265-266
simple carbohydrates, 120-121
Simplesse, 127
skating, in-line, 188
skiing, 188-189
skin, removing from poultry, 254
skipping meals, 104
slide aerobics classes, 185
Slim-Fast, 49
snacking
   solutions, 270-271
   teaching healthy eating habits to children, 27
sodium, reducing intake, 166-167
soluble fiber, 130-131
solutions

   for food cravings, 270
   for guilt, 40
   for negative thinking, 37-38
   for plateaus, 277-279
   for snacking, 270-271
   for weight maintenance, 279-280
soup recipes, 262
soy foods as protein sources, 123
spinning aerobics classes, 185
sports, 186
   burning calories, 189
   golf, 187
   in-line skating, 188
   skiing, 188-189
   swimming, 187-188
   tennis, 187
stages of change, 82-84
starvation mode, 20, 64
Steamed Vegetables with Herbs recipe, 266-268
steaming food, 258
step aerobics classes, 185
straight menu plan, 238-242
strength, effect of exercise, 179
Strength Log, 199
strength training, 178-179, 197-199
stress
   internal/external stressors, 223-224
   managing, 224-225
   psychological benefits of exercise, 178-179
stretching, 196
substitutes
   for fat, 127-128
   in desserts, 272
   low-fat food, 268
success, fear of, 229-230
sugar
   artificial sweeteners, 121-122
   effect on teeth, 166
   glucose, 120
   reducing intake, 165-166
   sources of, 166
   see also carbohydrates
sugar free, defined, 252
Sunette, 122
supermarkets
   canned food, 255-256
   dairy products, 253
   food labels, meanings of terms, 252
   frozen foods, 255

grains, 256
    meat department, 253-254
    Nutrition Facts labels, Daily
        Value information, 250
    poultry, 254
    produce department, 253
    seafood, 254-255
supplements, 136-137
support
    for do-it-yourself weight loss,
        76-77
    for weight loss, 230-231
    from family, friends, 30-31
    see also resources
support groups
    Overeaters Anonymous
        (OA), 65
    Take Off Pounds Sensibly
        (TOPS), 65
Supporters Worksheet, 76
Sweet 'N' Low (artificial sweet-
    ener), 122
swimming, 187-188

T

table manners, behavior modifi-
    cation, 213-214
t'ai chi, 178
Take Off Pounds Sensibly
    (TOPS), 65
teaching healthy eating habits to
    children, 27
teeth, effect of sugar, 166
tennis, 187
termination stage, 84
testing muscle strength, 198-199
thinking (negative thoughts)
    effect of, 36-37
    expecting perfection, 38
    solutions for, 37-38
thoughts (positive), 231-232
THRR (training heart rate range),
    196-197
to-do list for losing weight, 33
TOPS (Take Off Pounds
    Sensibly), 65
training heart rate range (THRR),
    196-197
traveling, eating habits, 273
treatment for eating disorders,
    43-44
trigger situations, avoiding, 82

Tufts University Diet & Nutrition
    Letter, 295
turkey, 254

U - V

U.S. Amateur Ballroom Dancers
    Association, 191
UCP2 gene, 28
University of California at
    Berkeley Wellness Letter, 295
utensils, basic kitchen equip-
    ment, 259
vegetable food group, 141-142
vegetables
    calorie/fat grams chart,
        285-286
    Creamy Vegetable Soup
        recipe, 262
    fresh, 163-164
    Janine D'Amato's Vegetarian
        BBQ-on-a-Bun recipe, 265
    shopping for, 253
    Steamed Vegetables with
        Herbs recipe, 266-268
    when to eat, 164
vegetarians, protein sources,
    123-124
very-low-calorie diets, 63-64
very-short-term goals, 84
videos (exercise), selecting, 193
Vinaigrette recipe, 262-263
visualization techniques, 214
visualizing serving sizes, 143-144
vitamins
    sources, 134-135, 160-162
    supplements, 136-137

W

waist-to-hip ratio, 17
walking
    burning calories, 202
    style of, 201-202
warm-up exercises, 181, 196
water
    alternatives to, 132-133
    drinking during exercise,
        176-177
    when to drink, 133
water soluble vitamins, 134

weather conditions, effect on
    exercise, 176-177
Web sites
    American Council on
        Exercise, 291
    American Dietetic Associa-
        tion, 291
    American Heart Association,
        292
    CyberDiet, 293
    FNIC (Food and Nutrition
        Information Center), 54
    Health Vision Diet & Weight
        Loss/Fitness Home Page, 293
    Healthtouch Online, 44
    Healthy Weight, 293
    Weight-Control Information
        Network (WIN), 292
weighing-in, 111-112
weight, *see* healthy weight,
    overweight people
Weight Change Chart, 111-112
weight cycling, 10-11
weight fluctuation, 111
weight gain
    compulsive overeating, 217
        questionnaire, 218
        solutions, 218-219
    differences among people, 21
    emotional responses, 21-22
    family influences on, 25-27
    from fat, 127
    reasons for, 20
    when extra pounds are okay,
        17-18
    yo-yo dieting, 10-11
weight loss
    alternative methods
        fasting, 56-57
        meditation, 56
    attitude toward, 82
        food avoidance, 214-215
        patience, 215
        visualization techniques,
            214
    commercial programs, 59-61
    commitment to, 207-208
    diet types, 48-50
    differences among people, 21
    difficulty of, 7-9
    do-it-yourself plans, 75
        evaluation questions, 77
        support for, 76-77
    effect of habits on, 18-19
    expectations, 40-41

expert advice, where to get, 53
fad diets, 20
finding information about, 23
goals, 31-32, 84-85
mixed messages about
    carbohydrates, 52-53
    counting calories, 51-52
    high protein diets, 52
    low fat diets, 51
motivation for, 68, 112-113
    alternative activities to
        eating, 113
    rewards, 114
number/size of fat cells, 19
personal assessment
    questions, 71-72
    eating habits, 72-73
    lifestyle changes, 72
personal attitude toward,
    68-71
preparation for, 81-82
    eating habits, tips for
        improving, 89-90
    exercise tips, 90
    motivation, 90-91
    stages of change, 82-84
recording, 111-112
resources for information
    books, 293-294
    magazines, 295
    newsletters, 294-295
    organizations, 291-292
successful strategies for, 12
support, 30-31, 230-231
to-do list, 33
yo-yo dieting, 10-11
Weight Loss Attitude Quiz, 68-71
weight loss plans, *see* diets
weight maintenance, 279-280
weight plateaus, 277-279
weight training, 178-179,
 197-199
Weight Watchers, 48, 61-62
Weight-Control Information
    Network (WIN), 292
Weight-Loss Challenges
    Checklist, 73
weight-loss support groups
    Overeaters Anonymous
        (OA), 65
    Take Off Pounds Sensibly
        (TOPS), 65
WIN (Weight-Control Informa-
    tion Network), 292

without added sugar, defined,
    252
women compared to men in
    weight loss, 19
workouts
    aerobic exercise, 195-197
        cool-downs, 197
        training heart rate,
            196-197
        warm-ups, 196
    cross-training, 200
    Exercise Log, 202
    schedules, 180-181
    strength training, 197-199
    walking, 201-202

Y - Z

yo-yo dieting, 10-11
yoga, 178
yogurt, calorie/fat grams
    chart, 287
Yogurt Vinaigrette recipe,
    262-263
Zone (The), 50

When You're Smart Enough to Know That You Don't Know It All

For all the ups and downs you're sure to encounter in life, The Complete Idiot's Guides give you down-to-earth answers and practical solutions.

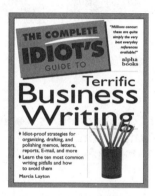
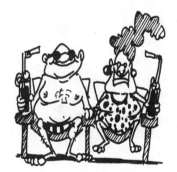
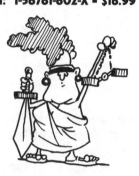
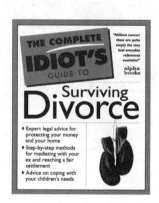

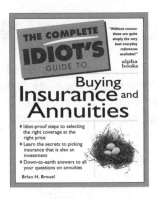
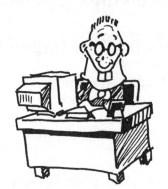
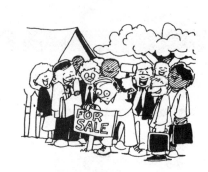
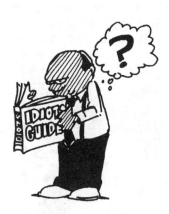
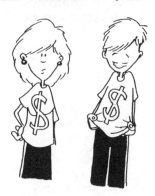
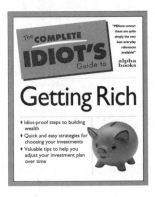

The Complete Idiot's Guide to Learning French on Your Own
ISBN: 0-02-861043-1 ▪ $16.95

The Complete Idiot's Guide to Dating
ISBN: 0-02-861052-0 ▪ $14.95

The Complete Idiot's Guide to Hiking and Camping
ISBN: 0-02-861100-4 ▪ $16.95

The Complete Idiot's Guide to Cooking Basics
ISBN: 1-56761-523-6 ▪ $16.99

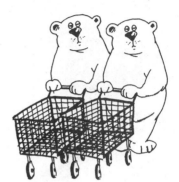

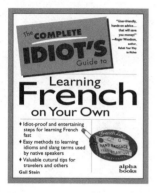

The Complete Idiot's Guide to Learning Spanish on Your Own
ISBN: 0-02-861040-7 ▪ $16.95

The Complete Idiot's Guide to Gambling Like a Pro
ISBN: 0-02-861102-0 ▪ $16.95

The Complete Idiot's Guide to Choosing, Training, and Raising a Dog
ISBN: 0-02-861098-9 ▪ $16.95

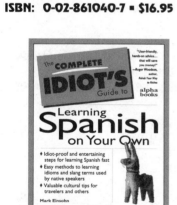

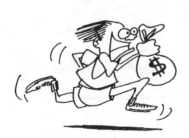

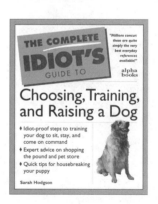

The Complete Idiot's Guide to Trouble-Free Car Care
ISBN: 0-02-861041-5 ▪ $16.95

The Complete Idiot's Guide to the Perfect Wedding
ISBN: 1-56761-532-5 ▪ $16.99

The Complete Idiot's Guide to Getting and Keeping Your Perfect Body
ISBN: 0-286105122 ▪ $16.99

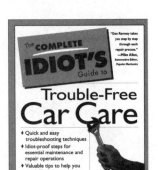
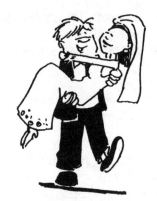
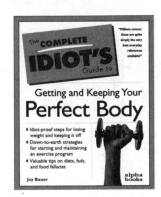

The Complete Idiot's Guide to First Aid Basics
ISBN: 0-02-861099-7 ▪ $16.95

The Complete Idiot's Guide to the Perfect Vacation
ISBN: 1-56761-531-7 ▪ $14.99

The Complete Idiot's Guide to Trouble-Free Home Repair
ISBN: 0-02-861042-3 ▪ $16.95

The Complete Idiot's Guide to Getting into College
ISBN: 1-56761-508-2 ▪ $14.95

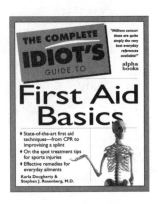
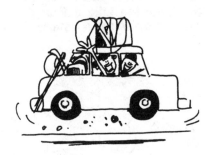
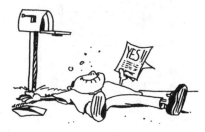

You can handle it!